THE BOY WHO FINALLY STOPPED WASHING

OCD FROM BOTH SIDES OF THE COUCH

John B.

Cooper Union Press

Published by   Cooper Union Press

This book was printed and bound by Bookmasters, Inc., Ashland, OH

Cover design by Ryan Feasel of Bookmasters, Inc.

                    Publisher's Cataloging-in-Publication
                      (Provided by Quality Books, Inc.)

B., John.
     The boy who finally stopped washing : OCD from both sides of the couch/
John B.
     p. cm.

     ISBN-13: 978-0-9791339-6-1
     ISBN-10: 0-9791339-6-3
     LCCN: 2007908028

     1.B., John--Mental health. 2. Obsessive-compulsive disorder--Patients--
Biography. 3. Psychotherapists--Biography. 4. Obsessive-compulsive
disorder--Treatment.
     I. Title.

          RC533.B15 2007   616.85'227'0092
                                    QBI07-600280

DEDICATION

To my parents who believed in me so that I could believe in myself.

To my wife who is able to calm me when the storm is brewing,
inspire me when inertia surfaces, and be with me under any circumstances.

To my children who unwittingly and effortlessly fill my life with joy.

DISCLAIMER

This book is sold with the understanding that the author and publisher are not providing psychiatric, psychological, medical, or other professional services to the reader. Please seek the help of a competent, experienced, and licensed OCD professional for such assistance.

Every effort has been made to ensure that the text is as complete and accurate as possible. However, there may be some typographical errors or mistakes in content. It might be possible that specific needs and circumstances for certain individuals may cause part of the material presented to be inappropriate. Therefore, the book should only be used as a general guide and not the ultimate source concerning OCD and its treatment.

The purpose of this book is to provide information only. No guarantees, either explicit or implicit, are made regarding the effectiveness of the therapies and approaches for any individual. Neither the author nor Cooper Union Press shall have liability or responsibility to any person or entity with respect to any loss or damage or any other problem caused, or alleged to have been caused, directly or indirectly, by the information contained in this book.

To protect the privacy of patients and others, all names of clients and any identifying material have been changed or omitted. Clients discussed are actually composites of several different sufferers. All possible efforts have been made to ensure the confidentiality of all clients.

QUOTES

Heisenberg's Uncertainty Principle: "The more precisely the position is determined, the less precisely the momentum is known in this instant, and vice versa."

Jesus Christ: "Don't worry about tomorrow; consider the lilies of the field and the birds of the air, they toil not yet they are taken care of by God, therefore we should not worry about what tomorrow brings . . ."

Abraham Lincoln: "I am slow to learn and slow to forget that which I have learned. My mind is like a piece of steel, very hard to scratch any thing on it and almost impossible after you get it there to rub it out."

ACKNOWLEDGEMENTS

There are many people to whom I wish to express my appreciation. First, I thank my parents for their inspiration and encouragement in writing this book. Without them, this book simply would not have been possible. They adopted and raised me, sacrificed for my treatment, took me to a psychiatrist when I asked to be taken, and did whatever it took to care for me. I am eternally grateful for the love, faith, hope and confidence they have always nurtured within me. I give them full credit for providing me the capacity to persist even when confronted with very difficult struggles. Furthermore, my parents are directly responsible for making me aware of the divine in everything. This knowledge alone provided sustenance for my journey.

My wife has consistently tolerated my bouts of high anxiety throughout the seventeen years we have known each other. She has listened to me and allowed me to see things through her eyes. Her tenderness, patience, and compassion have served as blessings to me. We will continue to grow and strengthen each other. Together with my parents, she gently encouraged me to write. She also typed most of the book.

I thank my friend Bob who played a vital role in helping me think carefully and critically about the development, contents, and the purpose of writing a book. I vividly remember gazing over the beautiful fall foilage at a restaurant in Harper's Ferry, West Virginia while we discussed the book. We talked about writing a book together, but we could not find a format that would be effective. He is a person who does what he says, a participant and not an observer. He had the belief in me to hand over the reins of the only OCD support group in northern Virginia after starting two groups that have helped thousands of sufferers and family members. Thanks to him, I met my supportive and talented boss.

The relationships forged and the insight gained from several therapists over the years have been critically important in shaping my thoughts about treatment. Sprinkled throughout the book is wisdom passed down by these healers. I cannot mention them all by name. I was very fortunate that my first psychiatrist in 1981, Howard, diagnosed me correctly and made me aware of the National Institutes of Mental Health research studies. Getting competent help early made a large impact on my ability to manage my OCD symptoms. He made two invaluable statements to me that have served me well over the years. He said, "You are in control of your behavior," (when I felt the OCD was in charge) and "OCD is not your fault, you did not ask for it (when I felt self-pity for my plight)." Special thanks goes to Joyce, one of my former therapists. She was a wonderful therapist who died a few years ago. I was very sad about her passing. She said something that still stays with me. She said, "Any problem that you have and deal with will make you a more understanding and compassionate therapist. Coming to terms with your insecurities and vulnerabilities brings a greater understanding of how difficult change can be and gives you a greater appreciation of change when it does occur."

My former and current clients, and the friends I made in the support group, have taught me an immeasurable amount about anxiety and life. I am honored to know these individuals who have experienced OCD. The bravest people are the ones who confront their demons. Keep fighting the good fight!

My colleagues have also played an instrumental role in assisting and encouraging me. My boss has been my mentor and had the belief in me to give me my start in the psychotherapeutic arena. His humor, guidance, genuineness, and practical assistance are very much appreciated. He coined the title of the book. In addition, he read the manuscript and made many suggestions about potential changes. My clinical supervisor has also lent immeasurable support and encouragement. She assisted me by proofreading my query letter that was sent to potential literary agents and publishers. She also read over the entire manuscript herself and provided invaluable feedback. With me, she spent more hours poring over the text and assisting me to edit the book. Her ideas about marketing were excellent. She and another colleague assisted me in self-publishing after I realized that the publishing companies were looking for a self-help book, and not a memoir. They took me step by step through the process. I owe them a debt of gratitude. Several other colleagues, too numerous to mention, have shaped the way I view OCD and anxiety as a practitioner, and I thank them one and all.

Barbara edited most of the manuscript two times. She believed in me from the very beginning, helping me feel more comfortable with writing about such revealing and personal information. She told me that she thought that the book had the potential to become a movie. She completely restructured the book, making it more organized and more readable. Before working with her, I was reluctant to divulge intimate information and other material that I had not deemed important.

My brother and father helped me with any computer problems that arose. Snafus proliferated, especially since I am not a skilled computer person. My assistants demonstrated the patience of Job, tolerating my technological deficiencies time and again. Without them, I would still be writing this book by hand with a feather and some ink. My father read through the entire manuscript and made suggestions that helped the grammar and the clarity of the book. He also spent countless hours assisting me in trying to find a publisher. His generosity will not be forgotten.

My mother and wife also read through the manuscript and made suggestions about changes.

TABLE OF CONTENTS

PREFACE

How did I finally stop washing? What's my secret? Even though the title suggests that I used to wash my hands frequently, I have never had a handwashing compulsion. However, I have suffered from the anxiety induced by scary, unacceptable, random, bizarre, and doubtful thoughts and their concomitant **covert** rituals for more than twenty-five years. I never began handwashing; therefore, it was not difficult to stop! **I improved by learning how to behave differently, thereby altering the way that my brain functioned!** Throughout my story, I explain the overall approach and what specific tactics and thoughts aided my progress. I do so from the perspective of both a sufferer and a therapist. The story will help illuminate and bring to life the disorder I know all too well.

The classical compulsive symptoms of washing, checking, and arranging, have been emphasized in the literature, often to the exclusion of experiences that are more familiar to millions of sufferers. Being an obsessive, internally compulsive guy, I wanted to highlight these unobserved manifestations of the disorder. Obsessive types have not received enough recognition and attention; I'm here to give it to them!

In this book, I will explore in-depth my obsessions and cognitive rituals (thoughts, not behaviors, that serve to reduce anxiety), including my current primary fear of being overresponsible for another's well-being. I am writing this book to give the sufferer a sense of what my thoughts, behaviors, coping skills, and strategies I employ are, and to show that it is possible to live a purposeful and fulfilling life in spite of Obsessive-Compulsive Disorder (OCD). It is a comprehensive examination of many facets of my life including relationships, family, school, and career. The book answers several questions: how does a person best respond to the struggle that is OCD?; how can a sufferer manage and tolerate OCD's anxiety during different developmental and life stages?; how can a person maximize his or her potential in spite of a disorder?; and what does the obsessive mind look like?

Consider this book a chronological continuation of my story in Dr. Judith Rapoport's best-selling 1989 book <u>The Boy Who Couldn't Stop Washing</u>. My name is Stanley in that book. My story begins in elementary school and ends at the very beginning of my college career. For those interested, Stanley appears in Chapter XVII ("Over and Over Again") on pages 129-132. I was twenty-two years old when the best-selling book was published, and now I am forty. I frequently wonder what happened to all the other sufferers whose stories comprised much of the text.

The Boy Who Couldn't Stop Washing explores my symptoms in a very brief and synoptic manner within a few pages; dozens of sufferers' stories and their main symptoms and treatment options are outlined in the book. The book served and continues to serve its purpose well by increasing awareness of OCD's prevalence in the general population, its phenomenology, its potency, and different treatment options. I recommend the book to all sufferers and their friends and families.

The Boy Who Finally Stopped Washing looks at broad topics and also probes the subtle details and intricacies of a life spent on both sides of the couch. The book completes my story until my mid-thirties and provides context to increase understanding of OCD. Each sufferer will probably find that he or she is walking in my footsteps at some (or many) points in the book. My book demonstrates the highs and lows of a person who has lived what appears to be a relatively normal and productive life to outsiders, but, in actuality is sometimes filled with pain and self-doubt. Since OCD is a part of who I am, I want to share my story about how everyday life influences the symptomatology of OCD and how OCD interacts with the demands of everyday life. I have attempted to keep a good attitude and a good sense of humor about my disorder and to remember that no matter how frequent, intense, or long an obsession lasts, I have the tools to manage my OCD when it flares up.

Though I possess the behavioral and biological tools to manage OCD, OCD has had a very significant impact on my life. Sometimes I have been emotionally exhausted by its incessant call for attention, and at times it has drained me of vital energy necessary for a happier, more focused, and less distressing life. It has even appeared to dictate, especially with soccer in my youth, which direction I have to take in life. I speak about soccer in my earlier years in Chapter 1 of this book.

I have been planning to write this book for at least twenty years. I feel very proud how I have confronted my OCD, my perfectionism, and my tendency to procrastinate without allowing the struggles to obstruct my life goals. That is what living with OCD is all about: persevering during the hard times, attempting and frequently succeeding in efforts to tolerate and manage symptoms, and appreciating life and its ups and downs whether symptoms are absent or very troubling. Remembering that high anxiety does not last forever, even though it may seem to, is a crucial piece of information. When one takes the hills and valleys in stride the majority of the time, faces life head-on without -- or with a minimum of -- avoidant and compulsive behavior, that person has mastered OCD.

The most difficult task while writing this book was to put the experience of OCD into words. The pain, the grip it holds on the sufferer, the intensity, interference, and the "life of its own" it inherently seems to possess are truly extraordinary emotional phenomena. During the ebb and flow of time, anxiety may swing from very high levels when a sufferer responds to false (anxiety) alarms in his or her nervous system (deer in the headlights phenomena), to times when the chaos has ended and a person is able to experience the world and all of its wonderful, terrible, awe-inspiring aspects. Energy can be channeled from unproductive, intrusive, and recurrent behaviors and thoughts to engaging in enjoyable activities.

In 1982, when I was a research participant at the National Institutes of Mental Health, I felt overwhelmed and suicidal. I spoke to Dr. Judith Rapoport, MD who evaluated me, and then I answered several questions from two more doctors. Next, all the psychiatrists, my parents, and I went to a large conference room to discuss my possible inclusion in the research study. After looking at the data, which included an overnight EEG, EKG, and a blood draw, the psychiatrists concluded that I did meet the criteria for the Anafranil (Chlorimipramine) study. One small part of that meeting stood out above the rest. One of the doctors discussed the typical course of OCD and my prognosis. He said that many sufferers led normal lives; however, many struggled to manage the symptoms at times in their lives. Life would be more difficult for me. After he said this, I dreaded my future and I hated him for being insensitive. I felt hopeless and at the mercy of pharmacological agents. However, I gained inspiration and strength from this encounter as the years passed. I promised myself that I would lead a normal life. I did not believe (or want to believe) that the doctor accurately predicted the days ahead. Over the years, I have come to be thankful for the doctor's truthfulness and bluntness. He provided grist for the mill that I always utilized whenever I envisioned a bleak, hopeless future; step by step, milestone by milestone, I was going to prove that I could thrive in spite of OCD and enjoy life to its fullest. Motivation and inspiration are essential when it comes to doing anything difficult.

I have learned many things about OCD personally and professionally over the years. I hope that the suggestions and conceptualizations will increase the sufferer's insight into OCD and, more importantly, help to modify maladaptive behavior. Feel free to use the suggestions and bits of advice that help. My recommendations do not specifically target every sufferers' symptoms because many have different thematic (washing, checking, arranging, fear of sinning, etc.) manifestations of OCD. However, with some creativity and insight, individuals can tailor strategies that reduce their symptoms. Regardless of the difference in symptoms and life situations, there can always be positive treatment outcomes. Psychotherapy (including insight-oriented and cognitive-behavioral therapy), my professional and personal education, and life experiences as a therapist and sufferer have helped me develop coping methods for others and myself. Please seek professional help regardless of making any gains using the suggestions in this book. A trusting, caring, supportive relationship with a professional is always a prerequisite for success using any therapeutic modality.

Related to the difficulty of elaborating upon my inner experiences is the apprehension that I feel revealing so much within this book. I made the very difficult decision to remain anonymous not because I wanted to, but because there were many personal and professional implications that this book could possibly have on my life if I decided to use my real name. I made the choice after much contemplation and reluctance.   I was determined to use my real name until others pointed out real consequences that could ensue because of using my name.   I don't want to change my relationships with any former, present, or future client, and I don't want the book to have a negative impact on my family.   Colleagues and family members made me aware of potential problems; I want to do whatever I possibly can to reduce the likelihood that anything negative even has a chance of occurring.

In spite of my decision, I still believe that openly describing OCD experiences is sometimes one of the only ways that mental illness will be destigmatized.   I am proud how much private material is contained within the book.   Thus, I am facing my fears and doing something I've wanted to do for many years.   Writing this book is the ultimate therapeutic act that I could have performed.

I was very fortunate to meet wonderful professionals very early in the course of my OCD; they were doctors who were on the cutting-edge of treatment.   I was diagnosed soon after the onset of OCD at age fourteen and given appropriate medication; medication that is still used today more than twenty-five years later.   I had a loving, caring, and sacrificing family that would do whatever it took to get me better.   And I was fortunate to have been geographically close to the leading experts in the field at the National Institutes of Mental Health (NIMH) where I met Dr. Judith Rapoport, MD.   Now I realize how much worse life could have been for me at age fourteen.   Without the presence of any one of the above professionals and institutions that directed me towards the most efficacious treatment path, my functioning likely would have suffered.

Here are some more experiences for which I am grateful.   In 1982, I took part in one of the very first research studies examining the effects of Anafranil (Chlorimipramine) on OCD subjects.   In the summer of 1985, I was employed in the NIMH department of child psychiatry.   Dr. Rapoport was the chief psychiatrist there at that time.   (Dr. Rapoport has played a pivotal role in my "OCD-life.")   I worked for the Anxiety Disorders Association of America for several months in 1990.   I met hundreds of people in an OCD support group that I led for five years.   I learned the inner-lives of the sufferers as traditional group boundaries disappeared while we socialized in restaurants, their homes, or elsewhere.

As a therapist, I have treated hundreds of people with OCD over a period of twelve years.   The disorder never ceases to fascinate me.   Sane people are driven to perform irrational, unreasonable, and excessive behaviors, and sometimes continue that pattern for years, sadly remaining prisoners of their anxiety even though efficacious treatments are available.

Fortunately, sufferers do not have to be imprisoned anymore. Medications are helpful for many, and cognitive-behavioral therapy (CBT) is beneficial for a large percentage of committed clients. I talk about these two empirically-proven modes of treatment later in the book. I had heard about the benefits of CBT for years, but now I know, after witnessing hundreds of individuals improve with psychological treatment, that this is a very powerful therapy. I have tried it myself and continue to practice it.

Before starting to read this book, the reader needs to know that there are two voices at work in the text of the book: the narrator's voice and my internal monologue. The internal monologue is set in italics and consists of my uncensored thoughts that are present in my mind at any given time. It is written in the present tense. The bulk of the text is written in the narrator's voice, mostly in the past tense, and tells the story and sets the stage for the internal voice. In addition, several places in the text, I have included entries from a journal that I wrote over the years beginning at about the age of fifteen.

The book is divided into three parts. In combination, Parts I and II are almost entirely in chronological order to increase the reader's comprehension and the book's cohesiveness. Part I "Growing Despite 'OC'stacles" describes experiences that occurred before I became a therapist. It begins with a look back at my story in The Boy Who Couldn't Stop Washing. I add more details to provide a fuller account. Part I finishes with observations about my wedding day. Part II "Years as a Therapist" commences with reflections about my wife's pregnancies, and explores the impact of OCD and the birth of my children on each other. The last chapter in Part II, "Review and Words of Wisdom," elaborates upon my growth as a person and my overall improvement in managing anxiety as an individual diagnosed with OCD. Part III, "Impact of OCD on Others" contains my wife's and parents' thoughts about how OCD has affected my relationships with them, and how I believe OCD has had an effect on my relationship with my wife.

Moreover, in order to practice what I preach, the words and phrases anxiety, fear, worry, scariness, bad feelings, nervousness, discomfort, and ruminations are used interchangeably in the text. I don't want to be compulsive and redundant with my word choices. Tension is used to denote a physiological response to an anxiety-inducing situation. Anxiety is used the most since OCD is an anxiety disorder. I frequently use the other aforementioned words during the description and implementation of treatment.

All names of individuals have been changed to protect their identities, and events, demographic information, and circumstances have also been disguised. The clients described are composites of several clients.

Hope is within reach. No, actually it is already embedded in each sufferer's heart waiting to be accessed. It is my hope that this book will aid the reader to discover the hope inside. For me, the concept of hope presupposes that something positive will come, we are just not sure when. Then there is more than hope with OCD; there is a way out of the OCD prison for each and every sufferer. All one has to do is allow oneself to do the things needed to improve.

.

PART: 1
GROWING DESPITE "OCstacles"

Chapter 1

THE BOY WHO COULDN'T STOP WASHING

In the best-selling book The Boy Who Couldn't Stop Washing, there are four pages about my years in school. However, some additional information and details would be helpful to gain a broader understanding of who I was as a younger person. A thorough investigation of the relationship between OCD and me is important. As renowned neurologist Oliver Sacks has noted, "To restore the human subject at the centre --- the suffering, afflicted, fighting, human subject --- we must deepen a case history to a narrative or tale; only then do we have a 'who' as well as a 'what,' a real person, a patient, in relation to disease."

I was in the fifth grade when I started to notice different and strange feelings and behaviors surfacing intermittently. The very first inkling or trace of OCD took place when I had to place my shoes in a particular spot on the floor for no apparent reason. The shoes had to be together "perfectly," the sides flush against each other, the toes making a straight line, and both shoes had to be perfectly parallel to the other without any protrusion of a toe or heel. Accomplishing all of OCD's rules required about five minutes. The momentum to act upon the discomfort built and crescendoed while I moved towards the floor. Then, upon completion of all the rules, relief reigned. I only did this ritual in my bedroom, therefore no one saw me go through all the steps.

The next inexplicable feelings of compelling anxiety happened when I was taking a state-mandated scantron test. These multiple-choice tests required the student to fill in a circle to designate the correct answer. I wanted to make sure that the electronic scanner gave me credit for each answer. Therefore, I spent excessive time ensuring that the circle was completely blackened, and that there were no marks located outside of the circle. The pencil marks had to be uniform; one part of the circle could not be darker than any other. The test was timed and I was extremely frustrated because I did not finish the entire test. In fact, I only finished one-third of it. I received a thirty percent, an appalling score for an A student. I didn't understand why I did so poorly. It eventually got chalked up to me not being a good test taker and being too perfectionistic. I was mad at myself because I should have done much better. I concluded that others were smarter taking tests than I was. I was too slow and slow meant "not as smart." I had no way of knowing at age ten what was going on; no one else did either in the 1970's.

Another symptom I experienced early on was needing to write using "perfect" penmanship. I had to make sure no words were touching each other, thus each distinct word was far apart from its neighbor, making reading a very arduous task. Also, I had to speak "perfectly," without any slips of the tongue, variations in speech, tone, or rate. Furthermore, my steps had to be in sync with my arms; everything had to be coordinated, which resulted in a robotic-like appearance. In fact, many variations in movement, no matter how subtle, triggered thoughts and feelings of inconsistency, disharmony, and doubt.

My awareness about defining my thoughts and behaviors as problematic due to some unknown force started in junior high school. I delivered a newspaper very early every morning. Having trained with other kids and getting help from my brother, sister, and parents provided me enough data to realize that there was something wrong with me. Nobody checked doors two or three times to make sure that a paper had been delivered. Looking back incessantly to see if papers had fallen off the cart was not a part of other's behavioral repertoire. Again, no one saw me, at least no one who mattered. I knew something was wrong and different, but I could not identify the problem. How was I going to talk to anybody about things that I didn't even know why I was doing?

The impact of my OCD was never more apparent than it was when I played soccer. I excelled at soccer and lived to play sports. But it was very difficult to cope with all the demands of being a good soccer player. I took things to heart more than my peers, like many of the kids that I have worked with whom have been diagnosed with OCD. (The typical profile of an OCD sufferer consists of traits including sensitivity and conscientiousness.) When I couldn't take the coach any longer, I quit. I cried while running around the field during practice for my all-star travel team. This man screamed at every little thing that he could. He seemed to derive pleasure from getting mad and throwing his weight around, taking out his life's fury on a smiling, innocent ten year-old boy. He made the game an awful, punishing experience; I began to anticipate getting nervous. I was nervous about becoming nervous. After my soccer coach yelled at me a few times, I didn't just quit that team, I did not play soccer on another team for the rest of my life.

My aversive experiences with this one individual were even that much more unpleasant on account of my inability to tolerate discomfort, personalizing what the coach said, and catastrophizing what he was screaming about. He wasn't targeting me, though it felt like he was when I was ten. And when he did yell my name, it was after yelling five other names. I was so anxious about attending practice that I could never say anything to my parents who might have given me words of encouragement and wisdom about how to handle this situation. I was paralyzed with fear. Nothing seemed to placate him. I believed my playing time would plummet each time he yelled, even though it never did.

He must have been extremely angry with me, disapproving of everything I was doing. I incorrectly concluded that he probably hated me.

Regrettably, my hypersensitivities, elevated levels of anxiety, and self-defeating ways of thinking about the circumstances I encountered caused me to leave a game I loved and a game at which I excelled. I practiced for hours and hours kicking and juggling a ball, and could juggle the ball three hundred times on my feet, knees, and head. I won juggling contests and referees often complimented me on great plays. I scored three goals in one game against an all-star travel team. I had inborn talent and skill and worked hard to improve all the time. One of my friends that I played with went on to play at Duke University and then played in the English Professional Football (Soccer) League. I stood out head and shoulders above my peers and had a promising future in the game.

Though highly-skilled, during games, I would lose myself in the OCD world of numbers. Two, four, six, and eight spun through my mind, trying to distract me from matters at hand. Indeed, concentrating on the mental chatter did cause blunders on my part, greatly increasing the probability that I would play uncharacteristically. But the more I tried to distract myself by being active, the more the obsessive thoughts bothered me.

Due to my internal focus, my teammates wondered aloud why I went through phases with seemingly little interest in a game. They yelled at me in frustration and didn't pass me the ball when I was unable to put the thoughts aside. Only when I could play with energy and vigor did my teammates treat me like usual. Of course, it made things worse when my peers were mad at me. I became anxious about what they thought about me and how my play affected the team. More anxiety led to an increased frequency of errors on the field; these in turn led to screaming by peers and coaches and higher levels of anxiety for me.

The beginning of high school saw a marked increase in severity, intensity, and duration of symptoms. One night I was lying on my bed trying to go to sleep. I could not turn off, no, I could not stop or slow down one iota the thoughts that went through my mind. This was the ninth or tenth day in a row that this had happened. They were the same thoughts and feelings over and over again. Persistent, intrusive, noxious internal experiences that simply did not change no matter what I did. Every time I heard my bones crack when I moved I had to count eight sets of eight. My bones seemed to crack with every movement at a joint. I was constantly cracking (up!). For some reason, the even numbers two, four, six, and eight were "good" numbers. Four would suffice sometimes for eight. Or four might be added to eight. In addition, if I did not say (to myself) the numbers correctly and adequately, I had to start all over again because I felt worse than when I started to count. It was a downward spiral that led me two times to freeze in front of others. I did not move because any movement might mean that bones would crack or my teeth might make noise. I was overwhelmed and couldn't talk about it.

OCD also impacted me tremendously when I was a member of a marching band and a symphonic band during my freshman and sophomore years of high school. I possessed natural ability in music, and although my OCD made practicing and performing difficult, I wanted to try to improve and do something I enjoyed. During one marching band competition, I was in the midst of an epic battle between falling into the seductive, illusory world of OCD numbers and the concentration necessary to know when to do what while I was marching in circles, diagonal lines, and vertical/horizontal lines with my clarinet. The big problem here was that both the music and the marching required counting to know when to start or stop. As you might guess, I occasionally lost track of what set of numbers were running through my mind and made small mistakes on the field. For example, in this particular competition, I was several steps from where I was supposed to be, conspicuously messing up. Another bad experience occurred during a symphonic band competition. I was so anxious that I couldn't play, read the music, or concentrate on what others were playing to get any perspective on where I was supposed to be in the music and how loud I was supposed to be playing.

Again, like my times in soccer, others did say mean things to me and about me. I felt terrible because my poor performances were affecting how others were evaluated. I stopped all band activities because it became too stressful and associated solely with negativity.

Two weeks after the "numbers" episode in my sophomore year in high school, I couldn't sleep one night. Numbers flooded my mind for an hour, making it very hard to sleep or do anything but to pay attention to this horrific mental thunderstorm. I realized that not everyone experienced such mental interference, and that apparently I could not do anything about it. I was in the ring with Mike Tyson, absorbing a merciless beating without any defenses or skills to block him. And maybe I needed help and should say something to my parents. No one else I knew complained about having intrusive thoughts and I had never had difficulty sleeping before all the numbers entered and consumed my brain.

So I went to my parents in the middle of the night, nervously revealing the distress that was keeping me awake. Though the numbers had appeared many times before, especially at night, I had always believed that they would soon go away. However, it was clear to me that they would not just disappear on their own. Furthermore, it was clear that my experiences were not normal; distress similar to this could not be typical. I couldn't explain it that well, but my parents took my angst seriously. I told them that I needed to go to a psychiatrist. I had never seen one; nevertheless, I knew the word. I probably didn't have knowledge of exactly what a psychiatrist did, but I must have been minimally cognizant of their role. I was very frightened to tell my parents about this bizarre stuff that I had in my head. I felt my heart sprinting when I told them. I didn't know what I had done to obtain and deserve such problems. The situation seemed hopeless and unchangeable. Insurmountable frustration was palpable in the room, leading me to pound my fist against the floor several times. Soon thereafter, my parents took me to a psychiatrist.

At approximately the same time the numbers and noises emerged as symptoms, I experienced an epiphany. There was more to girls than what I previously knew. I encountered the world of nude women through friends of mine who seemed to possess endless supplies of stimulating material. Meanwhile, my body was producing hormones at the normal, frighteningly high level of a teenager. I learned about self-stimulation and masturbated frequently to the pictures and images of beautiful, exposed women. My friends reinforced this behavior by making the materials available. An orgasm was extremely reinforcing, increasing the likelihood exponentially that my behavior would continue for the foreseeable future.

The worst thing about my awakening sexual appetite and awareness was the messy consequences. I was intensely focused on the clean-up after masturbating. I could not get clean enough and feared that others were aware that I had performed this behavior. I wondered what my parents would think about my actions. I spent hours attempting to reassure myself that all was clean, nobody smelled anything, and that, most importantly, nobody had seen me engage in the "unspeakable" act. I worried so much that I thought that I heard someone walking up the stairs to my room when no one really was. This reminded me of times when I had wondered whether I really heard a noise when I bent a joint. And I also wondered if the neighbors, on one side of the house closest to my bedroom window, had ever noticed me do the private act. I had noticed someone next door on top of their roof when they were working on it a few weeks earlier. How did I know for certain that there were no additional problems and that someone would not climb on the roof? How did I know if it was my anxiety influencing my perceptions or my perceptions reasonably increasing my anxiety? There was no way to be one hundred percent certain; the uncertainty was repugnant to me. However, I was not going to cease listening to my primal drives and hormones, which were screaming at me for release at this juncture.

On the other hand, I felt guilty about what I was doing and wished I could cut my penis off and die. How could something that didn't involve others and seemed to be the reasonable and obvious response when I had an erection cause this much distress? Why did my curtains and blinds never completely block out any neighbor's probing eyes? I obsessed very frequently about whether the neighbors saw me and if I should have felt guilty if they had. I knew that it was likely that no one had seen me. At that point in my development, I could not say, "So what . . ." to the "What if . . .?" question. I needed the correct answer, not just any answer, and I needed to know that absolutely and positively no one had seen me. I never felt like that.

The feeling of dread and horror reminded me of the time that my friend had opened a drawer in my bedroom and discovered my OCD journals. He read something about mental problems and asked me what it meant as I slammed the drawer shut. I made up a story but was shook up for days obsessing about the consequences of my peers possibly knowing about my troubles. It felt awful because I knew for certain that he had read something I did not want him to. I could not control what others thought and did, a reality that was distressing to live with.

Things did not get better as high school progressed. On September 15, 1982 at exactly 10:40 A.M., the "catch-up" game began. This was the time that the class ended.   Every movement, spoken word, personal thought and feeling of that moment is forever branded into my mind like an identification mark seared onto a cow. My mind was working overtime, and it simply could not "keep up" with every internal and external demand and stimulus. I entered a new psychological stage at that moment, a stage that lasted twenty years. My psychological world revolved around this one moment in time and a few very difficult OCD times that ensued. I referred back to this time several times each day, ruminating about the setting and the concomitant emotional chaos. It took twenty years before I did not refer to the distant past, and ten years before I didn't have an excessively negative emotional reaction to September 15, 1982.

September 15, 1982 was a school day at the beginning of my junior year in high school. I was fifteen years old. It was a day reminiscent of most days. Mrs. Hanford, my English teacher, was wrapping up the class and giving us homework assignments. I hurriedly wrote them down. Fellow students shuffled papers, quickly shut their books and binders, and some zipped up backpacks, preparing to dash to the lunchroom. Nobody wanted to wait one minute in the lunchroom line. Being an omnivore and a growing boy who was perpetually hungry, I also took to the blocks to commence the race down the hall.

To my right, high up above the classroom's front door, was a clock. It was one of those clocks that emitted a distinct and pronounced "click" when the minute hand moved. It seemed like the sound grew louder as the minutes ticked down to signal the end of class. Staring up at it, I noticed that the time was 10:37 A.M. Everyone was ordering his or her class ring during the lunch break and I had hoped that the necessary paperwork was filled out accurately. Free-floating anxiety saturated my entire being.

So much was happening in my life. I was worrying about the upcoming SATs, the difficulty of my classes, and most immediately and intensely about how I was going to buy the ring and eat lunch in thirty minutes. *It just isn't enough time! I barely have time to scarf down some fries on other days.   And can I be sure that the ring I am going to get is the one I want? Is it cool to purchase a ring? Is it effeminate?*

It all seemed to be too much; I couldn't process it all. OCD exploited my overwrought emotional state and it intensified and deepened in response. My books were organized and I resumed playing "watch-the-clock." *Where do I have to go to buy the ring? Did I measure my ring-size correctly? I've never owned any jewelry before. I better not mess up because it is really expensive and I'm paying for it. I wonder if my friends are buying rings and what will they think of mine?* There was so much required information on the form; I still was not certain about my ring-size since the measurer was so low-tech. *How am I going to get my homework completed tonight?*

Cccc. . .llll. . .iiii. . .cccc. . .kkkk!! My mind contracted and tightened when the minute hand struck the infamous time of 10:40 A.M. I couldn't keep up with my thoughts. They weren't racing thoughts, but intrusive, repetitive, distressing thoughts. Despite my internal processing problems, I bought the ring and did what I had to do. But the level of my anxiety skyrocketed to the point where there was nothing left to do to ward it off. Up to that minute in my life, I had always been able to "keep up" with and immediately ward off anxious thoughts and feelings. From that moment forward, until roughly the year 2002, I was trying to "catch up," to resolve feelings, thoughts, and events from the distant past.

Presently, I am not fixated on any particular event, thought, or feeling from the past. But, I speak frequently about some of my attempts to "catch up" and some events that became embossed and central in my mind in the following chapters. Typically, I am able to "let go" easier now. My coping is not perfect, but I attribute the positive change to maturity (finally, in my forties!!), life experience, OCD experience, and better understanding of coping with OCD in the face of everyday life. Now, I am the Duke of doubt, the Ruler of the relaxed, the Undersecretary of uncertainty, the Prince of (anti-)perfectionism, and the King of casual. Well, at least I am sometimes.

OCD is an extraordinary experience. Everyone sometimes thinks scary, disgusting, out-of-nowhere thoughts. For OCDers, whose brain functions differently and who have learned a behavior pattern of avoidance and compulsivity, the thoughts do not eventually lead to an internal peace, but provoke anxiety that can lead to rituals. OCD makes it much more likely that you will do a ritual (i.e., wash hands, think an opposite thought, think certain words in the "right" way, etc.) with the thoughts in order to preserve a fleeting "peace."

My high school proms and my college days are where this book begins. Most interesting to me are my days as a psychotherapist helping those with OCD and other anxiety disorders. Clearly, I have not been cured of OCD. However, I have learned how to manage and tolerate high levels of anxiety. No one can escape stress and anxiety; it is not humanly possible. The battles that individuals wage daily to protect and defend themselves against needless suffering appear to be winnable ones. They are. Yet the means of winning are different than many would expect. You must experience anxiety. This is an arduous task.

My chapter in The Boy Who Couldn't Stop Washing discussed very little concerning college other than the isolation, loneliness, and concomitant depression that I experienced due to my preoccupations with OCD. Entering my sophomore year, my symptoms began to emphasize and focus more on what others thought of me, not an unusual theme to be preoccupied about, especially for a young person. The difference for the OCD sufferer is the intensity, frequency, and duration of the anxiety associated with the uncomfortable thoughts. I became consumed with the anxiety and thoughts. Thoughts caused more anxiety and anxiety more thoughts, resulting in an ongoing, non-stop ride of sadness, lowered self-esteem, and increasing tension. Depressive episodes were not unusual.

The following is a story of decades of perseverance and persistence coping with OCD.

Chapter 2

<u>OC DESPAIR</u>

Late one night in the summer, I drove thirty miles home where some college buddies lived. We had a great time drinking a few beers and shooting the breeze. I was sober and needed to get home, but it was such a long ride. Going home, time passed at a snail's pace, lengthening my despair. It normally took about forty-five minutes to arrive home and I was all alone, trapped, and imprisoned in my car with my obsessive mind. My intricate internal world consumed and shielded me from my surroundings and most reasonable thinking. My Steve Winwood tapes, even when turned up ridiculously loud, didn't provide enough distraction, companionship, or solace. Songs about a "Higher Love" and "When You See a Chance (You Take It)" didn't ward off the barrage of negativity or make me feel better about myself. I was convinced that I would never experience any kind of romantic love. The music only reminded me of my loneliness and emptiness, there in the car and in my life.

Somehow willing myself to focus enough and just get home, I made it to my parent's house where I lived. My body and brain were numb; I didn't know what to feel. My body was at the house I grew up in, but my brain was back there on the road somewhere. *How did I arrive home alive tonight?* Despite all the suicidal thoughts that raced through my mind during the drive, I got there. I was shocked to find myself breathing, home, and in one piece. I wasn't sure if I wanted to be.

Revisiting the entire ride while leaving the car and entering the house, I realized that the most difficult part was taking that sharp curve on Turner Road. Part of me had wanted to continue going straight and plow into whatever was in the way. I was almost home, but was uncertain whether I could tolerate any more thoughts about harming myself. At that point, I really did not care what happened. I prayed for a safe return home, yet hoped for an "accidental" crash.

While getting ready to go to sleep, I began thinking more clearly about what had triggered all the suicidal thoughts. I knew that my life wasn't going exactly as I had planned. For optimal improvement, I wanted a girlfriend. I was happy with a nice, pretty girlfriend during the previous summer. The immature illusion, that all my problems would be solved if I only had a girlfriend, solidified and intensified. It was easier to think that my problems were external rather than needing to work on myself.

Lying down, I reflected upon the events on the road that night and I became extremely terrified at what had almost happened. I took pride in coping well with my problems. I believed that I was mentally tougher than the people who had attempted suicide. The events of the night humbled me. *Did something almost happen? Was I really that close to running into something? No, no matter how I felt, I would never run into or over anyone. At three o'clock in the morning there wasn't anybody on the roads anyways. Maybe I had hit an object on the road? Did I hear something suspicious on the road? Was it my old car complaining?* I couldn't be sure. Uncertainty is the hallmark of OCD, and OCD ran amok. I was certain about something; I was certainly uncertain.

Similar internal monologues tormented me continually. *I can't give myself that much time to obsess! I have never attempted suicide before, but why reach the point where I'm actually considering it? Was it something that I said? Or did one of my friends do something that triggered my depressed, obsessive, and ruminative state? No, I can't remember anything.*

Lying prone on the bed, not wanting to think about this subject for another second, but, nevertheless, feeling compelled to figure out if I had attempted suicide and why, I could not sleep. There's nothing better for an insomniac than a mixture of anxiety and depression. Ambien can't compete with this combination. *The car did go over the yellow line briefly. I must have tried to hurt or kill myself. Come on, every car that takes that corner goes over that line. It's a very sharp curve and I knew tonight that there weren't any other cars coming. Yeah, but what if a car was coming and what if I really did want to crash? The very act of crossing the line must have meant that I wanted to kill myself. It must be because I don't have a girlfriend. My friends do. My last girlfriend broke up with me. I felt so much better about myself when there was a lady around.* My level of depression was directly proportional to my level of anxiety.

Maybe the anxiety I felt about someone catching me "in the act" of masturbating also contributed to my depressed mood. I was uncertain whether my mother had seen me after I realized that the door was open a small crack two days before. Furthermore, the little amount of alcohol I had probably didn't help my depression. In deed, alcohol is an antidepressant.

I mentally revisited the whole drive home during the next week. I tried to remember every road I was on and every turn I took. *Everything's fine. No, it's not! The curve on Turner Road and the exit off of Jackson Highway have always been a problem. Look, John, I'm fine. I made it home all right. I did not hit anyone or anything because I would have known.* Though strongly compelled to do so, additional attempts at absolutely and definitively resolving whether I had hit anybody only made me feel worse. I knew that the next day would only bring something else to worry about. Another segment of the drive would violently and abruptly crash into my memory, waiting and expecting to be obsessed about. My mind functioned as an anxiety-magnet . Like a moth to light, I could not evade my fears.

A couple of days after the late night car ride, I began to obsess more about whether or not I truly wanted to kill myself that night, and, if so, might this horribly painful reality repeat itself. If it does not happen on the roads, then maybe somewhere else. The fear of going crazy and crashing the car symbolized a complete loss of control to me. I hated that feeling. *But remember, John, Dr. Smith said that I'm always in control of what I do.* From time to time, I got nervous around knives at home, fearing (but not believing) that I would hurt or kill myself. I knew that I was in control of my behavior; the heightened anxiety I felt when near a knife intensified near sharp objects. I perceived (it wasn't reality) that I had to exert energy to remain safe. The anxiety about hurting or killing myself wasn't new, but it was downright terrifying. I wanted to avoid both the kitchen and washing dishes because of my fear of cutting someone with a knife. I couldn't avoid eating, though meat could be "cut out" of my diet.

Of course, I did not <u>really</u> want to kill myself or even hurt myself that night on the road. A mixture of obsessive and depressive thoughts made it extremely laborious to feel good; painful inner experiences reflected how badly I had felt. Behind the wheel of a car was not the best place for me to be when I was feeling out of control of my life. I experienced the car driving me, and forces that were under my control no longer seemed to be. The car appeared to move even when I barely touched the wheel. I was just along for the ride; the car seemed to travel by instinct, turning onto roads with which it was familiar. I was confused, ambiguous, and uncertain about anything that I sensed or thought. *Who is in control of the car? I am, there is no one else here. Do I turn here? Is this the right exit? Sure it is. I always go there, but something looks different about it, right?* The conflagration elevated in intensity, and made a certainty appear very uncertain and almost wrong. Obviously, I was driving the car, however, my perception of the situation told me otherwise.

I despised the common insidious pairing of OCD and depression that I experienced in the car that frightful night. Alone, OCD was daunting. Together, depressive thoughts and ruminations only served to throw more fuel onto the emotionally raging fire. My depressed mind distorted my thinking and caused many situations to appear worse than t hey actually were. Sure, as previously stated, a girlfriend would have been nice, but she would not have solved all my problems. She could not eradicate OCD.

Thank God I don't think about suicide now. I don't know what helped me get through this dreadful car ride and its aftermath, but I pray that the strength continues to express itself. Most importantly, I hope to never experience that level of agony again.

Get help when suicidal thoughts start to creep into your consciousness. Get help immediately if plans for suicide develop and/or intention for it begins to emerge. OCD can stoke depression when a person already feels overwhelmed and helpless. Depression can increase the frequency, intensity, and duration of obsessions. High anxiety can cause subtle alterations in perception by increasing doubt. Approximately fifty percent of OCD sufferers experience at least one clinically significant depressive episode in their lifetimes. Fortunately, depression, like OCD, is also very treatable.

Regarding that awful night, one thing was clear. I **had** to learn different approaches and techniques to help myself with OCD and depression. I could not function with analogous internal experiences. Things had to get better; I could not continue living that way.

I was scared to look towards the future. It appeared bleak. But I knew that my life could only improve. I had always wondered what the future might hold with OCD. After the car incident, I used this curiosity as a motivator and an inspiration; I always wanted to believe that I would not be hampered by OCD. The doctors at NIMH five years before had stated that many people with OCD led normal lives. But they also pronounced that I would have OCD for the rest of my life. Thus, I was concurrently very curious and very reluctant to look ahead.

Chapter 3

SEXUAL OBSESSIONS

In the book The Boy Who Couldn't Stop Washing by Dr. Judith Rapoport, MD, one of the last manifestations that my OCD took was sexual in nature. By this, it meant that I obsessed about whether someone would discover that I had masturbated. Like all red-blooded boys, thoughts and images of beautiful women entered my mind, but sometimes I would obsess about whether these images were leading to too much self-stimulation. This chapter focuses on my anxieties about masturbating. Other chapters cover more material that explains my anxieties regarding additional sexually-based fears.

This is a subject that is difficult to discuss, but one that needs to be addressed in order to provide a full account of my life. There were very difficult times that occurred during my college days. Then, I took the subway with my father. We drove my car down to the parking lot and took the subway into the city. It would take a total of about forty-five minutes. On many occasions, there was at least one very beautiful woman sitting or standing nearby on the subway. Everyone was going to work; hence, the women were dressed elegantly and stylishly. Being eighteen or nineteen at the time, my hormones were at their peak. I might as well have been at the beach. I began to feel warm around these women and would get an erection. I clearly did not require Viagra then (and hopefully will not for some time). It was a very simple formula; gorgeous women caused erections. Moreover, it was the morning and I was not a morning person. Being tired increased the likelihood that I would get an erection.

I have always hated this about being a guy, not having control over my body. I remember sitting in the back seat on a long car ride when I was a teenager and worrying that someone might see me in such a predicament, particularly females. I did not want my mother or sister to see me with an erection, but I supposed that my father and brother would understand the discomfort. There was no controlling when I would get an erection. Well, I mean there was some control. If I intentionally looked at a beautiful woman in person or in a magazine, I would be likely to have an erection. But, I frequently had them when I really didn't want one. The more energy I exerted trying to deflate the culprit, the more helpless I felt.

The reason that I bring all this up (pun intended) is that it bothered me a lot --- a whole lot. Our sexuality and how we act on it is a very important defining characteristic. Like many adolescent boys, masturbating while looking at "girlie" magazines was very appealing to me, yet it was often an activity that led to much anxiety. Obsessions about whether or not everything was clean enough afterward, whether someone had seen me, and whether or not anyone could smell the evidence consumed me.

Another reason to be anxious, possessing the belief that I was performing an immoral act, originated from reading a religious pamphlet handed out at a subway station when I was thirteen. "Self-abuse" was the term used in lieu of masturbation. According to the material, masturbation was a sin and sexual stimulation of any kind should only exist for purposes of loving a monogamous partner or for procreation. Doubts persisted for years as a result of hearing contradictory information concerning masturbation. I believed that the culture around me sent irreconcilable messages about sex. Since my sexuality and sexual practices were central and defining characteristics, OCD found an emotionally significant "soft spot" that was already rife with chaos regarding sex in my adolescent brain.

I grew up in a middle class neighborhood and there was not much space in my bedroom. I had my own room, but it was very close to my brother's and not very far away from the stairs leading up to my room. Privacy was difficult and my anxiety soared in response to the close quarters. Someone could easily be within twelve steps and a closed door of me.

To make matters worse, since I was very young, my mother had always woke me up a couple of times during the night so that I would not wet the bed. I had wet my bed at least once virtually every night since I was a young child. She dutifully performed this task until I was approximately fourteen, certainly sacrificing much sleep over the years. Once, she found me with some "girlie" magazines underneath my pillow and I was very embarrassed. I wondered what she thought of my fascination with the female body and if her belief system viewed masturbation as a sin. I did not think so and had never heard her say so.

When I wanted to masturbate, I tried to wait for times when my anxiety was already low so that I could handle the rush of anxiety once it started arriving. My sexual drive or libido was stronger than the idea of evading such an anxiety-provoking activity. At night, I called out my brother's name, to see if he was asleep, so that I could feel comfortable masturbating. He was within twenty to thirty feet of me. In retrospect, the scant noise that I did make was exaggerated and out of proportion to reality, and seemed to me to be magnified one thousand times, just like all the other anxieties that I had suffered over the years. It was as if I had a small pimple on my cheek and believed that it was actually the size of Montana. That is what anxiety does --- it distorts, exaggerates, and magnifies. I can laugh at this now because the absurdity of it is evident. I also learned that masturbating is a natural, normal behavior that need not shame anyone.

It seemed that I often masturbated immediately preceding dinner. Not purposefully, but it seemed to be a pattern. I thought my family had some sort of strange sixth sense. No, not really, but I always walked down the stairs and washed my hands figuring that everyone knew what had transpired in the upper chambers. Of course, they didn't. I was sure they knew that I had masturbated since all boys did, and I was no different. Still, they could not have known each and every time it happened.

My anxiety increased the more I heard, or thought I heard, noises anywhere in the house. I have already mentioned that I often wondered if my brother could hear me. Sometimes I would stop masturbating and pretend nothing was happening, but I would usually manage to fight my way through this anxiety. The drive to complete the act was much stronger than the high anxiety associated with this very pleasurable activity. I heard footsteps when there were none; anxiety subtlely distorted my perceptions. But I continued despite my misgivings.

Speaking with my therapist helped me to put what was happening into perspective. He normalized my experience and helped me to laugh at myself. High levels of anxiety confused and disoriented me. I knew what was really occurring, but there was the obsessional static in the background. Elevated anxiety could also make normal feelings, urges, and behavior seem abnormal, wrong, and even immoral. As advised by my therapist, I told myself that even unbearable anxiety did not signal that I was doing something wrong. In the case of OCD, feelings were not facts and were frequently "false alarms" in response to a perceived danger. IT WAS NOT A <u>REAL</u> DANGER.

While in the grips of anxiety, different information infiltrated my mind and caused me to doubt the righteousness, or at least the acceptability, of masturbation. Intolerable anxiety emerged due to an overreaction of my nervous system to what it deemed to be potentially dangerous stimuli, in this case, other people who could possibly know what I was doing. So what if somebody knew? It would be very embarrassing, but life went on with or without others discovering me acting sexually.

Looking back into several OCD and life journals that I kept during my teenage and twenty-something years revealed some very interesting material regarding my struggle with sexual issues. It really helped me to remember some things that were very hard to recall, and it sparked much thought about my life. One very poignant vignette from 1985 described a time when my therapist recommended a very interesting, mysterious, and curious course of action. He wanted me to experience and learn that I was in control of all of my behavior, and that I indeed had free will and choice, even of my sexual behavior. He recommended that I walk to a nearby schoolyard at 2 A.M. and think about what was to occur there. I had to allow myself to understand how much control I really had in this situation. Upon arriving at the destination, my first mission was to find an area where there were several trees or bushes. After finding a hidden location, I was to touch myself in the crotch area of my pants. He called this exercise an "ordeal."

I thought that an alien had taken over my therapist's body and was saying anything to embarrass or humiliate me. *This is ridiculous! This will never work. What kind of recommendation is this? I'm not going to touch myself in public! I know it's two o'clock in the morning and probably no one will see me, but why do it?*

Inasmuch as I had developed a great deal of trust in my therapist, and nothing else had helped me deal with the tremendous amount of psychic pain that I experienced in response to masturbating, I tried his crazy scheme. And guess what happened? I learned that I was in control of my sexual behavior. No, I was not in charge of other's behavior, but I was in control of where, when, and how I masturbated. I had much more control of my sexual behavior than I previously believed. **I was in charge**. OCD had muddled my understanding of this very important idea. Humor entered the picture. I could even laugh at myself! Relaxation resulted when I had sexual thoughts, feelings, and physiological responses.

If I could orchestrate this entire scenario and carry through with it so early in the morning, I must still be in control of my actions. Before, my anxiety elevated so much when my hormones kicked in that it felt as if my own body was torturing me. If I could not extract those deleterious chemicals from my body, I had to coexist with them somehow. The absurdity of the therapeutic ordeal brought levity and perspective to a very distressing situation.

Learn to laugh at yourself. Most importantly, take recommendations seriously, even if they appear to be counterproductive. Trust in the therapist and the therapy and you will achieve better results in a more timely fashion. Reveal all your anxieties and disturbing experiences to your therapist so that he or she can best assist you.

Chapter 4

THE PROM NIGHT FROM HELL

Distressing sexual thoughts, including my fear of being discovered masturbating, continued. But, with insight attained through therapy, they were less potent and frequent. Nevertheless, masturbation was a subject to be educated about and even to embrace as part of the total human experience. Thoughts were just that, thoughts. Guilt generated by my mind concerning such matters was unnecessarily disturbing. My guilt decreased, too.

Then, my high school senior prom came. I was still a virgin and all I knew about the prom was that people drank in vast quantities and had sex. It often happened in that order, too. Sex became an issue that I was forced to cope with in-vivo and there was no way to escape it. Another person would play a part in my sexual life, though I realized that it was really only a date and not everyone really had sex. At least, I might have had to kiss a girl. A date, due to my inexperience with girls, appeared like a big deal. Kissing seemed like sex because it was foreign territory to me and it made me very nervous to contemplate.

My senior prom night was quickly approaching. It was supposed to be a very exciting time in my young life! But I was a very timid guy, and I asked the one girl that I really wanted to go with too late. She already had a date. She was a girl that I had a crush on since the ninth grade. I fantasized about her and was hoping, despite hanging out in different social circles, that she would say yes. I did not think that she would, but I had nothing to lose. Everyone went to the prom, or so it seemed. I had to at least ask someone, or I would be a total loser. It took me too long to build up the nerve. She was attractive and appealed to many guys who were not as reticent as I was.

During high school, my OCD was very strong and pervasive. Being almost constantly preoccupied didn't help make me the most outgoing person. Much of my energy was spent attempting to cope with OCD. Consequently, my social life suffered. It was so excruciating and painstaking to ask a girl for a date. Relationships with girls were problematic because I didn't possess the initiative and the self-confidence to speak much to them. I was average looking with an average build. I was not an athletic standout or an academic "superbrain." I was intelligent and earned good grades, but I was not part of the elite group of boys and girls who got straight A's every quarter and who took the most challenging classes. I told my therapist that I was a Rock with Impulses. He thought that this nickname was humorous, but was also an apt metaphorical description. I always thought, talked about, and looked (leered?) at girls and "girlie" magazines, but when it came to action, I was usually too self-conscious, sensitive, and anxious. Like a rock, I could only sit there. In the meantime, my hormones were coursing and percolating, unbeknownst to anyone, threatening my obsessive obscurity.

It turned out that a girl asked me out to a prom! It was someone who worked on the same floor at the bank as I did, was new in the area, and didn't know that many people. She wanted to go to her school's prom and the people who worked with us thought that the two of us would make a good couple. I was anxious and excited about the upcoming event.

Great, I was going to a prom, and I didn't care whether it was for another school and not mine. Everything was fine. I got the tuxedo, the corsage, and the flowers. I had a vague idea about where she lived, but I had never actually been there. I was so nervous about meeting her mother, having pictures taken, etc. I drove down the highway while looking to my right for an apartment complex. She lived next to the complex. My mind was racing, worst-case scenarios and notorious "What if . . .?" questions played over and over in my head. Every move that I made became micromanaged and overanalyzed. *I must be cool and calm. If I'm not, she won't like me.* My body and mind were stuck in fifth gear and I couldn't slow them down. I felt restless and shaky, as if I needed to jump out of my skin. I began to get a mild headache.

Oh, man. I missed the turn. What a stupid idiot! What does she think about me now? I missed the turn and it was right in front of me. How could I miss an entire apartment complex? Let me get over to the right so I can turn at the next road. It's not such a big deal. I've never been . . . man, did I stop at that stop sign? That guy was angry with me for going. Well, everything is OK. Why don't I just cut my losses and go home and say I got sick? I can't do this. My God, I can't do it! Am I going to kiss or hug her at the end of the night? Oh, here it is. Is this a space that I can park in? I don't know. She probably sees me looking confused. I may have caused an accident back there and I still don't know if I'm going to kiss her or not. Here I am. Let me go up and get her. What's everyone at the office going to think of me after tonight?

"Hi, Robbin. . . . Oh, hi Mrs. M. . . . Yes, we work together. Oh, I'm OK . . . . Oh, yeah, tonight will be fun."

Mrs. M. started taking pictures of Robbin and me, and I was still feeling very uncomfortable with the proceedings. My anxiety went so high that automatic pilot had taken over, and I went through the motions without really knowing why I did what I did. Exhaustion took over my mind; it did sometimes when all else seemed to fail. In hindsight, the context encountered there was new and different, and it was not surprising that I felt very awkward.

Finally, we were ready to leave. Her mother finished taking pictures and saying good-bye to us. Inconspicuously, I breathed a sigh of relief since we now had the green light to go ahead and escape Mrs. M.'s perceptions of me. *I'm alone with a girl I hardly know, and I have to drive us to the prom. This has never happened before. I'm a mess, too! Of course, it is a situation I want, but not here and not now. I'm sure my driving will scare her, and I have no doubt that we are going to have a lousy time . . . Oh, just shut up and drive!*

My resolve to keep fighting negative thoughts and anxiety was gradually giving way to the realization that it seemed that it didn't matter what I said to myself. My anxiety was sky-high and it didn't appear that it would drop anytime in the near future. It was one anxiety-provoking incident immediately after another; there was no chance to catch my breath. Anticipatory anxiety (anxiety experienced before an event or situation) about the prom washed over me and manifested itself by making me believe the worst would happen. I opened the car door for Robbin and then berated myself for not having pinned on her corsage in the apartment. *Her mother helped me! What must she think of me?* While thinking about that, I worried that her dress had gotten caught in the door when it closed, and that she might be mad at me. I was convinced that something horrific was really going to transpire.

Needless to say, my mind was incredibly unsettled and preoccupied. I could not focus on much of anything. On the way to the restaurant for dinner, I turned the wrong way on a street, going against traffic. Feeling stupid and embarrassed, I apologized repeatedly to help me settle down and to reassure her of her safety. It wasn't such a big deal with her because we were OK and had not crashed, but it was a huge blow to my ego, and especially to my belief that I was in charge of all my actions. I had the mistaken belief that OCD had caused my mistakes, and therefore, I was forever angry at OCD, cursing it every chance I got. It took a few years to learn that my angry reactions got me nowhere, and that having control of my behavior did not mean that I would never commit an error. Two to three years after the prom, and about the same time as my terrifying drive on Turner Rd., I ultimately realized that I had to learn to manage my own OCD. Things had to change. I could not manage and master something that continually upset me.

By now, I was so exhausted from worrying and obsessing that I paradoxically began to enjoy the evening. I allowed myself to be where I was with my current feelings, and I tried to pay attention to what was happening around me. *Feel and don't think so much.* We arrived and began eating and having an interesting conversation. I began to feel very good about myself for having a date and spending much time with her. I was not sure what the rest of the night would bring, or what either of our expectations were for how the night would play out, but right then, I felt as good as I could given the circumstances.

There were nuns supervising the event since it was a Catholic school. I had seen nuns before, but it felt very odd to be going to the party of my life with nuns in attendance. I started to question my integrity and motives whenever I did anything in their presence. I nipped these morality obsessions in the bud by identifying my thoughts as excessive and a sign of OCD. Robbin introduced me to her friends and we danced some. I hated dancing, particularly to fast, upbeat music. John Travolta I was not. I had three left feet, and I left them stomping all over Robbin's feet while I noticed others, anyone, glancing in our direction. I was extremely self-conscious; it seemed that a spotlight beamed on me as I took the floor. In reality, nobody could see me because the floor was so packed with people.

We were having a good time. The music, atmosphere, and company were good, and I was beginning to get a little more comfortable. Old thoughts were creeping back into my mind about the night's previous events and worries. I could brush some of them off, but others stuck like a fly to flypaper. Abraham Lincoln, my favorite president about whom I have read much, said it the best. He said that his mind was like a plate of steel, that once a mark was made on it, it was next to impossible to remove it. It was very difficult to create an imperfection, but once it was made, it was permanent. I could not resolve and feel right about going the wrong way on the road, but I could not stop and ponder this more, I had to keep going. However I looked at it, it still had occurred. I thought she would think that I was a real loser for doing such a klutzy thing. I believed that this one incident colored her perception of the entire evening and any other encounters we might ever have.

Robbin and I never dated again. I never knew if the mistakes I committed that night led her to think I was dangerous, untrustworthy, or in need of psychological help. I was aware that I was projecting some of my thoughts and feelings onto her, but I did not know how many. I responded in an excessively avoidant and diffident manner toward Robbin after the prom. My response made it very unlikely, no matter what she was actually thinking, that I could continue even a friendship with her. Girls made me nervous. I was a basket case. It was very hard to be cool when my brain overheated. In retrospect, after many successful outings with countless beautiful women (a slight exaggeration!!), I finally realized that my reactions to my mishaps were more important than the nature of my small, harmless mistakes. People were more forgiving than I thought. If I acted and thought more calmly, I felt more relaxed.

As stated at the beginning of the chapter, I did not plan to attend my high school prom despite my efforts to go with a girl I found very attractive. I was disappointed and discouraged, but not devastated by her response. *At least I won't have to be nervous around everyone. Dancing in public is nerve-wracking, and I won't need to be a great conversationalist, either.*

However, it was my last chance to go to my high school prom, and I was curious about all the excitement. Others got so energized and enthusiastic about the dance, and I wanted to understand why. It was primarily an evening of dining, dancing, and talking. It sounded somewhat boring to me. I probably misinterpreted some of my enthusiasm and desire to attend and mistook it for anxiety. Anxiety and (perceived) risk-taking excitement send similar signals to the brain. I tended to feel nervous because I lacked social confidence.

It was seven o'clock on my prom night, two weeks after the prom I had attended with Robbin, and I was thinking about the girl I had asked out at my school. *If only I had asked her earlier. Would she have gone out with me?* Unexpectedly, I received a phone call from my neighbor, Joan. We were friends and had been neighbors for several years. She told me that her sister Kim was crying uncontrollably on account of her prom date not showing up or calling. He was supposed to call her by six o'clock to make arrangements to pick her up. She wondered if I could take Kim to the prom so that she could go. Kim wanted to go since she was prepared and had spent a lot of time and money readying herself for the big night.

I was caught completely by surprise, but instinctively and reflexively I answered in the affirmative. I hated to see her so upset. And I could go to the prom that I wanted to go to anyways. I didn't have a tux, though. Where was I going to get one at this late hour? *No, what am I thinking? I can't go now. It's too late. The prom will start soon anyways. Why did I say yes? Now I have to follow through and at least attempt to find a tux. What have I gotten myself into? Why am I a nice guy who wants to make others happy? Yeah, she'll be happy, but I'll be an OCD wreck like last time.*

I called a local tuxedo store and told them about my dilemma. The employee joked about me waiting to the last minute to ask someone. He wondered why I had not asked someone earlier. I explained to him that I already went to one prom and my neighbor's date had stood her up. I wasn't planning on going, but I needed a tux immediately so that I could take her to the dance.

When I got to the store, there were three young male employees waiting to assist me. They were laughing about my situation and generally having fun with the circumstances in which I found myself. They were not being mean or rude, but I did feel extremely embarrassed and even a little humiliated. *They must believe that I'm a loser since I don't have a date for my prom. They probably think I'm lying about already going to one prom. Everyone who is anyone goes to his or her prom. They are laughing at my inability to do what guys do, to ask a girl for a date.* They hurriedly measured me like I was making a very fast pit-stop. I always hated males touching me (e.g. doctors), but this was too much. Two guys were taking measurements simultaneously, one of them looped a tape measure around my waist and the other measured my inseam. I felt like an object that could not, despite my insecurities, do anything to protect itself from these intrusive workers who were touching me near (it seemed like it) sensitive, private areas. I feared that I enjoyed their hands touching my clothes that rubbed against my skin, and I kept reminding myself that I hated guys doing this. I knew that they were only doing their jobs. The fear returned in rapid-fire succession because they had to touch me more in order to ensure accurate measurements. I needed a tux, and they were simply helping me. Someone had to help me. I knew this, but I was humiliated and anxious, and moreover, anxious about my feelings of humiliation and embarrassment. I was obsessing about obsessing, a sure sign that I was overreacting and overthinking.

After acting like a madman to get a suitable tux quickly, I rushed back home. With the tux already on, I hurried next door. Before I knew it, Kim and I were a couple and her father and my parents were taking pictures of us. We were placing flowers on each other and generally feeling good about what was to transpire that night. *We're going to the prom and there won't be any nuns there.* Speaking of flowers, I became extremely anxious about pinning the flower on Kim's chest. She had large breasts and I had always noticed and appreciated her figure. These sexual thoughts frightened me and I compensated by not wanting to brush up against her inadvertently. Being The Rock With Impulses, and a hormonal teenager, I was that much more aware of the conflict between having to complete this time-honored tradition despite my high level of anxiety, and my fantasy world which would have made me rip everything off of her. Individuals with OCD are frequently over-controlled in certain domains of life; I would be the last person to do anything unseemly, bizarre, or salacious. And of course, all that happened was that someone else helped her with the corsage after witnessing my awkwardness and inexperience. Everything was fine. I had lived many years that spilled over with desires, randy thoughts, overly-controlled behavior, and anxiety about whether or not I could contain myself when in the proximity of a sexually desirable woman. That night, I passed the test with flying colors.

We were just friends anyways. We went with another couple that included one of her friends and her friend's brother. It was the most relaxed situation that anyone could possibly have wanted, no one was attempting to make any grand impressions and conversation flowed comfortably. Nevertheless, it was anxiety-provoking because I wondered how I fit in and how I was performing as a substitute date. *Do others really accept Kim as my date and am I earning any guy points for showing up with a female? Do my peers think more highly of me because I arrived with her?* I had competing feelings about remaining at the event. I was curious to see what the night held and how much fun I could have. However, since I had virtually no history of dating or partying during high school, I was extremely anxious. I had a hard time knowing what to do or say. I was completely out of my element and in unfamiliar surroundings. Plus, I felt very scattered and numbed by all that had transpired that evening. Feelings of embarrassment remained with me throughout the evening, though I enjoyed myself for most of it.

I mentally revisited the tuxedo store frequently during the evening. I was still trying to reassure myself that nothing occurred at the store that I did not want to have happen. The act of reassuring assisted the OCD to grow stronger. Self-reassurance is a common strategy, or ritual, that individuals use to reduce anxiety. For anxiety management, it is important to generate anxiety so that one can learn to habituate, or desensitize, to it.

We did not stay at the prom much longer. My anxiety decreased as we exited. The four of us went to a local all-night restaurant and ate. The only thing left was the good-bye kiss. My mind could not feel right about it. *But we're only friends. Do I just peck her on the cheek or hug her? The guy needs to be the one to initiate any action and appear confident. I don't know what to do!!! And my anxiety is making it more difficult to think about how to say good night. It's manly, isn't it, to kiss the girl? But we're only friends, remember? Who really cares what happens. I don't know what to do, so I will let her dictate what happens. I guess this is alright.* Doubt persisted. I made it through the innocuous, unremarkable, and anticlimactic departure from Kim with minimal emotional damage. She simply came forward in a hugging posture and I reciprocated. Easy. My anticipatory anxiety was much higher than the level I felt when the feared incident actually occurred. Anticipatory anxiety usually functions this way. I made it through the evening without making a fool of myself, and OCD did not negatively impact my experience.

I did not let OCD negatively impact my experience by distracting me or consuming me to the point that I was not as aware of my surroundings. I was determined not to permit anxiety to run rampant as it had during the first prom. It was present and that was OK. When I felt OCD surfacing, I paid more attention to the experience of my senses. I tried to remain in the moment, in the here-and-now. Let the anxiety flow and participate fully with the environment, experiencing all aspects of it. Remind yourself that no matter what you are thinking or feeling, behaving in helpful ways is the most powerful means of feeling happier, more relaxed, and in touch with the present. Dating more is a great way to help anxiety when you are actually on a date.

Cognitive changes are also very useful. My attitude was very negative about being with a girl and about expecting the worst to happen during the first prom. Clearly, by challenging some of my underlying assumptions concerning being with a girl, I could have injected reason and reduced my anxiety by examining all the evidence that I had accumulated. I had not dated much and had never had a terrible, forgettable night-out with a girl. I was imagining the worst when the best was just as possible; I discounted positive experiences and possibilities.

My anxiety fueled negativity. But I could do something about the anxiety **and** the negativity. If the anxiety was aroused by unreasonable, irrational core assumptions and beliefs, I could challenge the thoughts. For example, at the two proms, I talked to myself using a lot of shoulds. I told myself that I should (must, have to) do this or I should say that. Excessive "shoulding on myself" resulted in a rigid and moralistic outlook on what was right and wrong. Shoulds made me feel guilty when I did not have to. I also thought in catastrophic terms, making the worst outcome the most likely one to occur. I could not do something because then she would think badly of me and would never want to see me again, or there was **no possibility** of something good coming from my actions. Only terrible, unthinkable consequences could ensue from my actions. Thinking is something that everyone has some control over. Internally, speak differently and more rationally to yourself. This is another strategy that assists one through such trying times. The goal is to change the irrational thoughts that unnecessarily increase anxiety, not to self-reassure and reduce anxiety when OCD themes are present. For instance, in the case above, I eventually learned to utilize cognitive-based techniques to help me think more rationally about what has and what is likely to occur when I was with a woman. Armed with healthier thinking, I was then more capable of confronting my fear of making a fool of myself head-on.

Chapter 5

SELF-SABOTAGE

The most frustrating thing about OCD for many others and me is that although we follow the disorder's rigid rules, we still have to pay a steep price. In other words, in carrying out compulsions that reduce anxiety (including overt or mental repeating, counting, revisiting, and listing), one does not get the satisfaction that typically results from one's efforts. I may feel OK and be less anxious, but I am working with great diligence and not receiving a great payoff. Even though it is not therapeutic, the seductive force of the obsession attracts me. I find myself thinking that I must do or think something to decrease discomfort (compulsion), and so I do it. But, then I get annoyed because unlike a usual situation where a reward follows from work, soon after avoiding the anxiety or engaging in a compulsion, I will be back where I started. The very brief and temporary respite from high anxiety results in additional obsessions and compulsive behaviors, and therefore a vicious cycle continues. No matter what you might think to the contrary, OCD rules are not advantageous to follow.

The most obvious example of setting myself up to fail that comes to mind is when I used to tell myself during my undergraduate years, "OK, I'm going to look at the clock and then everything will be all right." Before performing this "magic," I felt anxious, uncomfortable, and out of kilter. As a result, I created the ritual of looking at the clock to eliminate all "bad" feelings and be in a new "good" state of mind. You can guess how long that lasted. That's right -- about a minute. At any rate, I had a minute, . . . a minute that consisted of no obsessing about anything before this break in time occurred. How long are humans able to completely and totally control their thoughts? A very short time indeed, especially if one is suppressing thoughts and distracting him or herself from feelings. Trying to control thoughts is counterproductive.

I was engaging in magical thinking, carefully watching the clock and hoping that everything was going to change and be great. Of course, this was not rational. I knew it wasn't, but I thought it wouldn't hurt to try, especially since I was in tremendous emotional distress. *What do I have to lose*? The illusion of a never-ending peace grabbed me and shook me forcefully because I continued to believe that if only I did it "right," I would somehow be rewarded. All the past obsessions, worries, and anxieties, including the 1982 incident and other "distant" anxieties, would disappear, and I would be left with peace of mind and tranquility. The notion that it could be possible to erase obsessions of events that occurred years previously was very enticing. *If only I do it "just right."* Whatever "just right" meant was not clear to me, but I felt it. But OCD found a way to torment me even more. I only had one chance to get it "just right," and that one time was exactly at midnight. Sometimes I wouldn't get it right and would wait for 12:01 A.M. to get it "just right." Emotional comfort was a mirage that disappeared when I approached it in this way.

Doing it "right" is very important to OCD sufferers. Individuals go to extremes to assure themselves that they have performed an act correctly, thoroughly, and perfectly. In the "clock watching" situation, I actually called the phone company to hear when the top of the hour was. Using the tone on the telephone as a cue for peace to follow, and disquiet to vacate, was a compulsion. On the other end of the line it said, "At the tone, the time will be 11:59 and fifty seconds, beep . . . at the tone, the time will be 12:00 o'clock exactly . . . beep." I liked the notion that the time was exact. It even said it was. Not much in this world is so exquisitely precise; there is even an "atomic clock" to make certain it is so. Everyone in my time zone heard the exact same message that I heard. People in other states and countries heard another tone and message, but it was just as correct for their time zone. This tone synchronizes the entire world, truly being the only thing that everyone has in common besides our human genetic heritage and basic survival needs.

My mother saw me watching the clock one evening and inquired about my fascination with it. She had no idea what the purpose of my actions was. I told her the truth. I didn't like to tell my parents too much of this craziness, but she caught me. *I can tell her, she's my mother. She already knows almost everything anyway.* Her reaction was very comforting. It was not reassuring in the OCD anxiety-reduction sense; her response did not directly target my fear and decrease anxiety. It was reassurance that was not a ritual. She was not attempting to specifically decrease my anxiety and strengthen my OCD. She said, "I'd probably do the same thing if I thought that it would work to alleviate my internal pain." What a great thing to say! She did not want to see me continue, but she conveyed a general sense of understanding that was very warming and supportive to hear.

Likewise, I attempted to resolve all my problems "magically" by starting fresh at the beginning of the year. Like most, reflecting, pondering, and planning for the future are activities that are performed around the time of the New Year. People's best intentions of changing are reflected in their New Year's resolutions. It is such a natural time to think, and perhaps act on the behaviors that you would like to eliminate, modify, or add to your repertoire. For me, it's no different. In years past, my OCD compelled me to live up to such a high personal standard of behavior that I was losing ground. Not necessarily a high moral standard of behavior, but behavior that I previously contemplated changing or adding in some subtle, nuanced, and perfectionistic way.

For example, right at the stroke of midnight, I would attempt to "snap-out" of any obsession and feel happy and content. Everything had to be "perfect" and "completely and thoroughly enjoyable." Again, feelings and thoughts were required to be "good." I could not make a false move or say something without assuring myself that it was an intelligent statement or inquiry. I was trying to become perfection incarnate.

Pressure mounted as the minutes passed by. I wanted so much to escape uncomfortable feelings and thoughts. I expended tremendous amounts of energy trying to satisfy my OCD. Being in this "perfect" state of mind required that when I performed a task for the second time, it needed to be precisely like the first time. No variations were permitted. Symmetry between the same behaviors became important.

As I'm sure one could guess, my feelings of "forced bliss" at the beginning of the New Year lasted about one minute. It was like feeding my compulsivity a big steak, thereby strengthening the urge to experience life in a robotic and constrained manner. But after that minute, the temptation for total and eternal emotional calmness (elusive and impossible) subsided. I knew that I had to return to living life in all its beauty and ugliness. On some level, I had to acknowledge that I could be perfectly imperfect like everyone else.

One day, still during my undergraduate days, my psychiatrist and I discussed the topic of how, so many times, I had set myself up to fail. It was good and useful to have goals and want to help myself. On the other hand, I had to be realistic about what I was pursuing. I was attempting to wipe the slate clean and rid myself of any unpleasantries. Of course, this was never rational thinking. It was all-or-nothing, black-and-white thinking that was common among OCD sufferers. Using this thinking makes the world a dichotomous place where no gray, in-between area exists. Everything is extremely one way or completely the opposite. Anxiety drove my irrational thoughts and actions, and anxiety and a misunderstanding of the nature of thoughts and feelings perpetuated the cycle. The more I tried to hold back a thought or a feeling (which is often a result of an irrational underlying thought pattern), the more the thought or feeling presented itself. In short, suppression, inhibition, and avoidance led to more frequent thinking about the very ideas and images from which I was attempting to escape.

My psychiatrist went on, stating that discomfort was a part of life. Emotional suffering was a normal and necessary part of life. Yes, necessary, if one wanted to lead a full and happy life that included others. Trying to avoid uncomfortable feelings set a person up for failure, and was akin to evading any pangs of hunger, experiencing the pressure of a full bladder, or contracting any viruses or illnesses; one couldn't escape any of them. A full life was only possible when some discomfort was present at times.

I believe that reacting in a more accepting, tolerant manner to discomfort is the most adaptive way to cope with uncomfortable feelings.

Expecting a certain amount of uneasiness and unsettledness helps to lower the impact of suffering when it surfaces. Of course, one is not attempting to bring pain onto him or herself unnecessarily or masochistically. (I'm not speaking about generating anxiety for therapeutic purposes. I will talk about that later in the book.) However, when discomfort occurs, one will be ready for it and not completely taken by surprise. An essential skill is to experience a full range of emotions, making the goal of being a genuine, authentic person attainable.

Another way that people set themselves up to fail occurs in cognitive-behavioral therapy (CBT). Exposure-response prevention (E/RP) is the specific form of CBT that treats OCD. The therapist works with the client to achieve a course of steady progression. Slow progression is fine only when treatment does not grind to a complete halt. To ascertain whether treatment is moving along or heading toward stagnation is a judgment call by the therapist. It is very sad and distressing for me to treat a person who doesn't stick it out in therapy. I know that they have reasons, which to them seem to be good ones, to want to cease therapy or to be satisfied with an incomplete recovery. However, I also know that CBT works. It has worked for me and for millions of others. With insufficient treatment, sufferers stop before confronting the stimuli (objects, thoughts, images, etc.) that are more anxiety-producing. Something is scary and the flight response activates. It is an evolutionary tendency that has served humans well throughout history. Yet, in this instance, it is unfortunate.

The client's reaction can frustrate therapists and leave clients half-treated. Half-treated people tend to revert back to old habits. OCD is like a fungus; if it is not thoroughly addressed, it will tend to grow back and spread.

Sufferers sometimes believe that once they begin to experience some freedom from symptoms that they "shouldn't feel any OCD ever again." They forget that the course of OCD is a waxing and waning one. They are going to have times, perhaps many times, when they revisit or think about engaging in an old pattern of behavior. The notion that they should never relive something that is believed to be resolved is irrational. We cannot control all that we think. But, OCD sufferers do have control over how they behave. They may need some assistance with motivation and need to become educated about the function of anxiety and rituals in their lives. No one has to continue to shower for an hour or more a day or wash his or her hands excessively. Nobody has anything on his or her birth certificate that identifies one as a lifelong compulsive bather and washer.

I say most of this elsewhere in the book, but it does bear repeating, particularly in the context of this chapter. There are only two empirically-proven ways to treat OCD. There is no reliable evidence that indicates that any other form of "treatment" is efficacious in attacking and reducing OCD symptoms. Any other "treatment" will result in self-sabotage. The first effective modality targets the symptoms cognitively and behaviorally, asking sufferers to adjust gradually to increased levels of anxiety. The astounding thing to be aware of about CBT is that this form of therapy, like medication, changes brain functioning. **Brain chemistry alters in an OCD client who has**

improved with CBT alone; research demonstrated this at the NIMH. The second effective modality, pharmacotherapy, is a useful and sometimes necessary component of the treatment regimen. Many professionals believe that the ideal treatment for most individuals suffering from OCD consists of both therapeutic modes. I agree with this assessment, remembering that some people do not require any medication. Keep in mind that some OCD sufferers are also diagnosed with an additional disorder(s) that may complicate the treatment picture – such as depression, a different anxiety disorder, or a personality disorder, just to name a few. These may require different types of treatment.

Unfortunately, there are other forms of "treatment" that mental health practitioners offer for OCD. None constitute real OCD treatment and they undermine a person's ability to get better. Some of the modes of "treatment" include insight-oriented therapy, psychoanalysis, and other talk therapies. If you are sitting in a chair or lying down on a couch for months or years at a time talking about your OCD symptoms, and figuring out the causes of the symptoms, you are not being treated for OCD. You are being treated for depression, low self-esteem, getting along better with others, or some other diagnosis or difficulty of living, but you are not being treated for OCD symptoms.

So often, I hear terrible, tragic stories about people who have experienced years of some other form of therapy before arriving at the door of a CBT therapist or psychiatrist who is knowledgeable in the treatment of OCD. This results in the waste of thousands of dollars, years worth of time and energy, ongoing symptomatology, and mounting frustration and anger with the entire mental health establishment. I hate to see this happen, but I understand why it does. Most professional people --- whether nurses, social workers, psychologists, or psychiatrists --- receive little or no training in CBT. Well, OK, they may learn about Pavlov's dog along with everyone else and think that CBT is simplistic and superficial; maybe scientists dressed in white coats in laboratories devise it. All I know is that it works, and it often does in a matter of months rather than years. I know it does because I have incorporated its principles in the self-management of symptoms, and in the successful treatment of many patients with whom I have worked over the years.

Participating in an OCD self-help support group does not constitute treatment, but it can be very useful for those who suffer from OCD. I led a support group for five years and greatly appreciate the role that they do play as an adjunct to CBT and/or psychotropics. Sufferers do not feel alone and they attain a sense of belonging and connection with others in a safe, non-judgmental environment. Participants can also learn more effective coping strategies. Check your local newspapers and call your local mental health association for information regarding groups. It is a fantastic experience to discover that you are not the only one to suffer with OCD, and that others have a deep emotional understanding, not solely a rational understanding, about your distress.

Twelve-step OCD programs can also be very helpful for some. However, relinquishing control to a higher power does not appeal to some people in our secular world. Furthermore, OCD does not lead to an addictive state like the one illegal substances do in better-known twelve-step AA programs. There is no pleasure gained when washing your hands over and over again. Pain and distress permeate the act.

Be aware, if you are not taking an SSRI (selective serotonin reuptake-inhibiting) medication (e.g. Prozac, Luvox, Paxil, Zoloft, etc.) and/or being treated with CBT, you are not receiving OCD treatment. It is imperative that people remember this!

Despite the many pitfalls obtaining efficacious treatment, there are some steps that   greatly increase the likelihood of success: find an experienced and knowledgeable therapist and/or psychiatrist; select professionals that one feels comfortable with and trusts; and receive empirically-proven treatment that is affordable. People change everyday. Of course, they must want to change and **act to change**, and not only wish that a positive transformation occur. Family members need to learn how to assist the sufferer. This support includes not reassuring them or performing any behavior that reduces the sufferer's anxiety. Also, the family can encourage the sufferer to take medication or seek CBT.

One of the most difficult hurdles to overcome in OCD treatment happens when a sufferer's natural and usual manner of interacting with others, and their typical way of solving everyday problems are pathological. A few sufferers come to believe that their symptoms are justified, and that others should make any necessary accommodations to help them get through the rough times, the OCD road bumps. It's not their problem if they can't get out of the shower; instead, it's somebody else's fault for not helping them get out of the shower in the first place. These same individuals may believe (and not only feel) that others should shower longer and use an entire bar of soap each time. Not only is OCD present, but also a maladaptive value and belief system that often sabotage treatment, making anxiety-generating treatment much more difficult to get them to do since they do not believe they or anyone else should do certain things.

I am describing one of the most common personality disorders associated with OCD; it is OCPD (Obsessive-Compulsive Personality Disorder). Righteous rigidity, pervasive perfectionism, strict stinginess, and a dearth of expressed emotion are some primary characteristics of a person that is diagnosed with OCPD. Someone with OCPD, unlike OCD, is not distressed about his or her behavior, or his or her value and belief system, either. He or she is distressed by anxiety and/or depression because of being very troubled by others' reactions to his or her rigidity. A crisis life situation (e.g. loss of job, divorce, etc.) can also cause great discomfort and lead them to treatment.

The individual diagnosed with OCD and co-morbid OCPD is more difficult to treat than someone with OCD alone. The world-view of an OCPD individual consists of fundamental beliefs and values that oppose and cause great difficulty in performing casual, relaxed, and flexible behavior. Hoarding, excessive acquiring and the inability to organize and discard objects, is currently defined as a manifestation of OCD. However, hoarders are predisposed to possess many more OCPD characteristics and are therefore harder to treat. (In the near future, hoarding may not be considered OCD behavior.) Having OCPD can be an obstacle to OCD treatment. However, despite difficulties because of the presence of a personality disorder, the person can still make gains that will lead to a happier life if they want to change.

OCD sufferers who also have OCPD can become very powerful, intimidating, and domineering people. The combination of anxiety-driven OCD behavior together with a rigid OCPD belief system and world-view can sometimes result in inappropriately expressed anger or in rare circumstances can even lead to aggression. (Please, do not confuse OCD with OCPD. Hollywood is one of the biggest culprits. There is only a one-letter difference between the two; however, the nature and origins of the two disorders couldn't be further apart.) Because of the intimidation and the need for harmony in the family, family members do what the OCPD person wants and run to their aid. What people understandably and naturally do in these circumstances is often exactly what is least helpful to the sufferer.

Family members must find a way to tolerate some backlash from the sufferer. If they can't, the treatment will be compromised. I frequently recommend that family members seek supportive therapy with another therapist to resist impulses to soothe and comfort their family member. Sometimes family members take me up on this suggestion; these families as a whole are better equipped to help the OCD sufferers. Emphasizing the importance of the familial context in which the sufferer lives, I even suggest that if the family is strapped financially, I will take a hiatus with the sufferer's treatment (often talking to the client for a few minutes on a weekly basis by telephone to assess his or her current situation and how he or she is reacting to the family's change of behavior) until the family receives the help they need. This is how critical family help is. Most of the families I have met need some support. Not because they lack intelligence or ability, or they are to blame for their loved one's condition, but because anyone living with an OCD sufferer needs assistance in knowing how to handle certain situations. Family members sometimes unwittingly and unintentionally reinforce compulsive behaviors.

Chapter 6

FINDING ME OUT

Since I typically have not engaged in overt rituals, most people who know me have been surprised to find out that I have had to deal with OCD. There have only been a few times in my life that it was obvious to others that something was awry. Those times took place when I was a teenager who did not have the skills that I now possess to manage OCD. I was overwhelmed by obsessions and compulsions; the phenomenon of intrusive, recurrent, and undesired thoughts was new to me.

I've always prided myself in hiding my obsessions and compulsions from others by fitting in and not standing out. My friends might remark in jest that I always stand out for some reason or other! I have always been amazed at what I can do while the obsessive background noise and pain try to interfere in my "other" life. I'm leading two lives, an inner and an outer one. This is particularly true when my anxiety is high.

An example of my intense desire to keep going and not be discovered despite being anxious happened the night before my graduation from college at a bar with some friends. I was with some friends having fun on a weekend night. I went to the bathroom, and then worried that my zipper was undone as I left. No, not just a little worry, but a worry that slaps you, a worry that you are forced to pay attention to and maybe do something about. Despite remembering that I had zipped up, my OCD wanted me to double and triple-check by returning to the bathroom. At that point, I said to myself that I was there to have fun with my friends, and that was what I was going to do. I was not going to be preoccupied and/or return to the bathroom quickly. They would wonder why a guy would do that. So I ended up enjoying myself by soaking up my surroundings; the obsession did not resurface in a potent manner. Of course, the thought was there, but if I could just keep talking, drinking, looking at girls, laughing, telling jokes, and being more outgoing than usual, I could get my mind off of the bothersome thought. It worked that night. Sometimes it does and sometimes it doesn't. Distraction is a good self-management technique for

OCD, but it is not going to assist you with decreasing the frequency and intensity of your symptoms in the long run.

There have only been a very few places where I wondered if someone could "read my mind," if they knew somehow that I had some mental static to attend to. One of these places was at a graduate school internship where I worked in the inner city. I worked with the chronically mentally ill, most of whom had spent many years at inpatient hospitals.

My supervisor was a very intelligent, hard-working and caring woman. I learned a lot from her and remember and still utilize some of the lessons that she shared with me. A requirement of the internship was that I needed a certain number of hours per week of supervision. Supervision involved talking with an experienced clinical social worker about the individuals that I was assigned to. Supervision also consisted of learning more about myself so that my awareness heightened about the effects of my behavior on an individual in therapy.

Well, this last point was the one that got to me. I loved to learn about myself, yet I was not so sure about the venue. *What if she can tell that there is more to me than meets the eye? There is with everyone, what are you talking about? No, if anyone can tell that there is some extra stuff going on in my head, wouldn't an experienced therapist be the one who would notice? They get paid for listening and observing behavior.*

Every time I left her office, thoughts of her wondering whether I was not fit to be in the social work field entered my mind. I felt unsettled and uneasy. I didn't like the way these supervision sessions were going; they seemed more like my own personal therapy sessions rather than discussions about others. I knew that it was important to know more about myself, but I had been in therapy for ten years already and thought that I knew myself well enough.

Then, one day she said what I feared. Well, not exactly, but close enough. She observed that at times it appeared that my attention was pulled away from her onto something else. *Oh, my God! She is on to me. She knows more than she is revealing. She knows that I have OCD.* She attributed my inattentiveness to me thinking about what had just been said and not listening to the current words. She was very perceptive. She was absolutely right. There was no getting around it. Many obsessions and compulsions intruded upon my mind and distracted me from the flow of conversation from time to time. A mixture of thoughts about what had already been said, together with my OCD thoughts, made listening closely in the present a big struggle. I suffered from OCD; of course, this was going to happen.

I left her office convinced that I was never going to make it as a social worker, and especially not as a psychotherapist. My anxiety was so high that the normal process of walking down the stairs, getting into my car, and driving home took on a surrealistic feel. I was so preoccupied with thoughts about having to leave the profession that the stairs and the cars around me were not quite in focus. My mind concentrated only on her comments and observations. Everything was a blur. I kept telling myself that no one could read my mind.

She can only see my external behavior and say something about that; she doesn't know what actually is occurring in my head. Therapists can't read minds. There was no way to know what she truly believed and observed. I chewed on this all the way home and for the next week. I had dreamed for many years of helping others with OCD, and now I believed that my chosen career path was in jeopardy because of the darn OCD, the very disorder I wanted to help others with.

My anxiety and uncertainty about her knowledge of my disorder or any other problem, and the ensuing doubt about my adequacy and competence to be an individual who could be effective working with others, remained high. During the same week, my anxiety elevated even more when a member of a therapy group, that I was a participant in, announced that she would not want a therapist who possessed any doubts about his or her abilities. Needless to say, this bothered me quite a bit. However, I knew that my anxiety was really related to OCD uncertainties and not to professional competence. For I had received very positive feedback from clients, other students, professors, and even my supervisor. It took some time, but, as always, as I proceeded in my training, my persistent discomfort diminished. I was able to take a step back and gain perspective on the situation while still remaining at the internship site with the same supervisor. Repeated times in supervision, and taking what she had said about my inattentiveness and learning about my behavior, were key elements that assisted me to recover from my fear. Speaking to my wife and my psychotherapist didn't hurt either.

A situation that could have left me reeling for some time also occurred in graduate school. It was another time when I obsessed about whether someone knew I had OCD. In one class, the professor, who himself was not a CBT-oriented therapist or teacher, was teaching about cognitive therapy and CBT. He was talking about treatment in general, not treatment of OCD. Cognitive therapy focuses on automatic negative cognitions and the rational, reasonable rebuttals and replacement thoughts that can lead to greater happiness and positive behavior change. He also discussed CBT, explaining how this therapy uses the precepts from cognitive therapy, but also targets undesirable behaviors for extinction or reduction in frequency, intensity, and duration. In OCD, both distorted cognitions and avoidant or compulsive behaviors serve the function of decreasing anxiety. Changing OCD behaviors will allow thoughts and feelings to follow that are congruent with the desired, more adaptive, non-OCD behavior.

I knew a lot about CBT and decided to talk in front of the entire class to educate them about it. I did not mention my struggle with OCD or how I had gained knowledge about CBT. However, I did make a remark that precipitated an OCD episode. Near the beginning of the presentation, I reported to the group, "I lead a self-help support group." During the remainder of the presentation, I was preoccupied with the precise meaning of that statement. I struggled with my own thoughts while I continued defining and describing CBT. *Did I just reveal myself? What if these people now know that I have OCD? I did say that it was a "self-help" group. Who else besides a sufferer would attend such a group?* After obsessing for a while, I told myself, "Maybe they know, maybe they don't." It was a cryptic statement and not a direct, intentional disclosure. *I said it and I don't care how people react to it. So what?* I reminded myself that many individuals who become therapists have dealt with their own issues over the years. *This is a bunch of progressive thinking people. I don't care what they think about me! So what! Even if they know I have OCD, they will not hold it against me.* I had never thought anything else so liberating in my entire life. The talk went well, and I was extremely proud to have managed this difficult episode so well. Of course, no one mentioned anything about my "disclosure," and no one treated me any differently after that class. *Being uncertain is not so bad after all.* Over the years, I have often used "So what?" as a helpful response to "What if . . .?"

As a psychotherapist, I occasionally wonder if my clients pick up any clues that suggest that I might have OCD. I honestly don't think that OCD impacts on my work or is evident in my interactions with clients. I don't do any rituals that would give me away and expose my diagnostic identity. Times when I process information a little slower than usual (because of an excessive amount to process) are apparently not obvious to others. I learned from my clinical supervisor that I had to attend to the conversation, no matter what. Fortunately, when I'm in a session, even when my OCD is bothering me, I am always able to concentrate on what is transpiring. However, my concern about my OCD becoming visible does heighten from time to time, especially when I empathize with sufferers, commenting on what they are experiencing in vivid detail. Sufferers typically nod, smile, and agree with my elaboration, without realizing that I really do know what they are going through. *But they don't know I have OCD, either.*

It is clear to me that I have become more comfortable as a sufferer helping others who suffer with the same disorder. As I have developed my own style and gained experience, I know that others, despite what I think, believe that I fully comprehend OCD based on my professional qualifications. My understanding of the topic is expected and essential to positive treatment outcome. Individuals do not automatically assume that my knowledge of OCD indicates any personal experience on my part. Though, from time to time, that is what my OCD would like me to believe.

Chapter 7

HYPERSENSITIVITIES

My self-consciousness, sensitivity, and doubts have at times left me vulnerable to put downs. I remember one incident when I was in my fraternity house after finishing final exams as a senior in 1988. I was lying down relaxing on one of the couches in the main area of the first floor of the house. A fraternity brother walked in and said, "What are you doing there?" I was in a relaxed daze at this point and said, "Resting, I just finished my last exam and I'm real tired." He replied, "John, go somewhere else to lie down, stop being a homo." He was out of the room at that point and I was too tired to respond. I didn't say anything; something that might have lessened my obsessive response to the statement. My brain immediately grabbed at this incident and made it mine. I obsessed about it for two years, replaying it over and over in my head dozens of times each day, frantically attempting to resolve the obsessive puzzle. It became one of my "distant" obsessions since it lasted so long. There was no way to disprove completely that he did not mean what he said, thus the doubt and uncertainty remained. I have always been a very sensitive person, easily hurt by the verbal whims of others. Despite my attempts to reassure myself that he didn't mean what he said, and that all was well in my world, this exchange persisted in my mind. It was not all right with me. And there didn't seem to be anything I could do about it.

After this incident, I kept wondering if I was gay. This guy called many people "homo" when he was goofing around or upset about something. He probably even doubted his own sexuality on some level. Even though he was just joking around and decompressing at final examination time, I took him seriously. I began to wonder if I **really** was gay. Doubt set in even though I had never been with a man, never wanted to be with a man, never dated a man, or done anything but the "normal" guy things with my buddies. I was never attracted to a man in a sexual way. I knew gay people and I believed that they deserved the same rights I had. I was not against homosexuality, and the non-OCD part of me knew I liked women. I dated women, had had sex with a woman, and couldn't take my eyes off attractive women. I was afflicted with chronic stiff neck from watching the world like it was a tennis game, ogling and leering at attractive women as inconspicuously and dignified a way as possible. As soon as that fraternity brother made his flippant, silly, offhand remark, an obsessive switch turned on in my head. Frequent thoughts and doubts entered my mind, turning everyday activities into a constant struggle to maintain my psychological and sexual identities. *What would it mean if I even glanced at a man? What if I happened to blink my eyes at the same time a guy's face showed itself on the television screen? What would it mean if I approached a man for an unrelated reason; couldn't I even ask for help in a department store for crying out loud?* I was tortured at every turn.

The fraternity brother had caught me at a very vulnerable time. It was during finals in my senior year of college. I was exhausted, not having slept one bit the night before. Thoughts of mitochondria and Aristotle's syllogisms intruded and crowded out my typical thoughts, and I felt more defenseless and out of control of my own mind, not to mention what was impinging upon me from my surroundings. Furthermore, my life seemed headed in a vague, dark, and unknown direction; did I like science enough to attend medical school or did I want to work for a year and take my time to decide? And if I chose to work, where could I get a job with merely a psychology degree? Everyone had earned one of those. My head swam with uncertainties and possibilities.

An added concern was that perhaps this one incident reflected the truth of my relationship to the fraternity at large. I tried hard to fit in with the northerners from New York, New Jersey, Massachusetts, and the like. Maybe when they imitated a local disc jockey saying, "Get her boy!," and asking if I had performed any Dukes of Hazzard stunts over the weekend in my very old, run-down, 1975 Plymouth Valiant, they were insulting me rather than simply having fun with me. I didn't have the cash, the car, or the pedigree. Maybe I was only the disrespected fraternity mascot. Worst of all, since graduation day rapidly approached, I wouldn't see most of my fraternity brothers ever again. The last thing my fraternity brother and perhaps others nearby experienced was him saying that I was a "homo." I wouldn't be able to show them that I was a cool guy anymore. Nor would I be able to defend myself or discover if the way I was interpreting their behavior was reflective of reality.

I have always been a quiet, reserved, and an externally casual guy. Early on, awkwardness and inhibition defined my relationships with girls. A few times over the years, a peer would intimate that my timidity and lack of bravado suggested that I was gay. It didn't happen very often, but when it did occur, I didn't understand it and was horrified by his or her assessment. But I knew that I was not targeted any more for teasing than other boys. Starting in the sixth grade, feelings I had when I was near girls made it clear that I was attracted to them. Then, the epiphany that I experienced at the age of twelve, leafing through "girlie" magazines with my buddies, was amazing. I knew at that moment that I liked what I saw and that I was as straight as an arrow. But doubt persisted back at the fraternity house.

My fear of being homosexual and the concomitant fear that others might think that I was gay were excruciating and torturous. I couldn't go anywhere or do anything without doubting my sexual orientation. I knew that my uncertainty was totally and completely unfounded. But, I couldn't shake this thought. It would not go away. I could not escape the doubt.

In order to fend off these fiendish thoughts and emotions, I approached very beautiful women. I didn't realize it at the time, but looking back on it now, I think that I rationalized that attempting to date very attractive women must mean that I was straight. Sure, I got rejected a lot, but I didn't have anything to lose. Maybe one of them would say yes, validating what I knew the entire time anyways.

Thankfully, I didn't pump myself up with male hormones or try out for a porn movie to "prove" my masculinity. I didn't do anything crazy in response to my distress. I just allowed the obsession to run its course. More truthfully, the obsession ran its own course. I remember reassuring myself frequently, telling myself that I was straight. As I've stated a few times already, that behavior served only short-term goals and was not helpful in the long run. Reassurance only served to reinforce the fear. What I really needed to do was to invite the anxiety in and experience life, and not avoid any event or interaction because of my anxiety. In fact, I had learned that it was important to induce anxiety in order to help myself recover from OCD. One exercise I tried was that when I watched television, I blinked at a man on the screen, and then held my fixed gaze on him so I could see him if he blinked back at me. This exposure to anxiety was repugnant, but it was effective in confronting and managing my obsessive fears. My staring behavior was part of an exposure strategy. I will elaborate upon exposure therapy, or as it is fully known, exposure-response prevention therapy (E/RP), later in the book.

For the next several months, my OCD symptoms exploited my sensitive temperament, and made it difficult to let go of even the most mildly pejorative words from others. It was as though these words catapulted literally from someone's mouth into my ears, and then they found their way into a part of my brain that allowed them to stick and remain for a while. My reaction to the offhand remark expanded my fears; I was not solely fearful of homosexuality and others thinking that I was gay. Before my mid-twenties, I pressed onward with numerous anxieties about what others thought of me.

Conditions have progressively improved in terms of defending and sticking up for myself when my initial reaction might be to agree with someone else's negative assessment. I used to go along with what other people said and take it as the truth. Now, I am aware when I start to think that way and I challenge those self-defeating cognitions. Of course, now I realize that my word and judgments are just as good as anyone else's. Whenever I found myself saying negative things about myself, I challenged those thoughts with statements to myself like, "I have handled this type of situation before even when I was anxious, I know I can do it again," and "I didn't ask for OCD just like a diabetic didn't request diabetes." *This is a tough disorder to cope with. I have to stop trying to make everything OK in my mind, and live with some anxiety and uncertainty. Come get me, anxiety, hit me with your best shot. Is that the best you can do?*

There are many more examples that demonstrate my extreme sensitivity to others' words. In the Preface, I said that as a young boy, I didn't want to let my teammates down. When I was up to bat, I remember being very scared of the spotlight in which I found myself. There was just too much going on around me and swirling inside of me to attempt to hit a ball; I cried about striking out. Even though I was an excellent soccer player, I messed up in this sport, too. Of course, messing up was very subjective and I catastrophized by thinking that if I struck out in baseball or missed a penalty kick in soccer, that meant that everyone would hate me and I was terrible at the sport.

After graduation, I was involved with initiating new members into the fraternity. It was a great honor for me to assist in this endeavor because it seemed so cool to me. At that point in my life, I did not have much money. I was working at a retail store after I graduated and did not need any nice dress clothes on the job. In fact, I did not have the money for new suits and ties. Upon arriving at the fraternity house, I talked to a few of the brothers and prepared myself for my part in the festivities. It was almost my turn to start. "Just a few more minutes," someone said. Another brother walked by, stopped, and began speaking to me. Then he said, "That's a nice suit, John," in a very facetious, insulting, and condescending manner. Being a guy who became very nervous when someone said something that might have been a minor slight against me, this indisputable pejorative remark hit me hard. It pierced me as the "homo" remark had. I did not know what to do, so I did not do much. Rather than respond in a fight or flight fashion, I froze. As he walked away, I stood there stunned and listless, confused by the entire incident. I felt a cold wave of dread, fright, and uncertainty wash up my spine and move into my head. I could do nothing but accept what had happened. I felt completely and utterly defenseless against the enormous force of the emotional blow; someone that I knew had rejected me. It seemed to validate what I had feared about my reputation at the fraternity. I surmised that if he felt this way, others must, too. My greatest fear had come to pass and I could do nothing to erase what had transpired. The very worst consequence was just beginning to become evident to me. At that moment, I knew something, and I knew it as well as anyone could know anything. This event was going to stay with me for a long time. A certain kind of defeatist, pessimistic feeling enveloped me as it had in the past. For the next two years I obsessed about this incident, reliving and replaying every excruciatingly painful moment of the entire experience. I obsessed about it and the gay theme simultaneously. I felt as though I had not done enough to help myself and had let myself down by not managing and tolerating the onslaught well. I beat myself up over the incident.

Thankfully, there were several months during my undergraduate days that were almost OCD-free. These days were a few months before the negative fraternity experiences happened. I had started dating more. My confidence (and hormone) levels were higher than ever. I was a brother of a great fraternity and had a very active social life. The possibility of becoming a doctor and all that it implied --- being able to help others, feeling fulfilled, and financial security --- were looming on the horizon. These days were months ahead of my negativistic and scared outlook right before graduation. A beautiful, intelligent, and sophisticated blond woman was a part of my life. All the pieces of my life were in place. In addition, the medication Chlorimipramine (Anafranil) I was receiving from England helped decrease my anxiety very significantly. I finally felt free from ruminating and obsessing about the past as much.

During the good times, there were too many positive aspects and too much structure in my life to spend my time OCDing. What a wonderful, liberating time it was not to have to think about and feel negatively about something that happened years before! Sometimes, the things that would have bothered me before only rolled off my back and bounced off my chest. My mind didn't seem to need or gravitate to grabbing hold of an incident and squeezing it until every drop of blood drained from it. I was not as sensitive to any perceived and real slights and did not care excessively about what others thought of me. The difference in how I felt was amazing to me. That was the first time in my life that I truly realized just how much OCD had been negatively impacting my life. I have always believed that individuals who have never suffered OCD will never completely appreciate the power of the experience. Perhaps it is not possible to fully understand something that one has not experienced directly. For instance, I do not understand what it is like to have diabetes, epilepsy, or to be a war veteran.

Most people have a built-in mechanism to help them reestablish psychological equilibrium. This mechanism was functioning better for me during my good undergraduate times. Things that people said rolled off my back. The mechanism helps people when they get extremely anxious about something happening, and more importantly, to cope with the consequences and implications of that occurrence. During my difficult undergraduate days, my anxiety about the gay theme and displeasing others created a mental atmosphere that made it hard for me to envision the whole picture, and to think of reasonable rationales to use in my self-defense. I was left speechless. I didn't practice assertiveness and standing up for myself.

Another type of experience that can lead me to become quagmired in OCD quicksand and leave me in a vulnerable state (when I'm hypersensitive) occurs when I feel bad about something, and this results in obsessing about feeling bad. Anxiety consumes me, especially when I feel vulnerable and sensitive. I remember a picture that a therapist showed me years ago that illustrates what happens to a person as anxiety appears and increases exponentially. The outline of one person did not contain the word <u>anxiety</u>

inside him or her, representing a calm person. The more anxious the person became, the more words were inside the body. There were several depictions of bodies that devolved until the last one was entirely covered and completely filled with the word anxiety. The individual was entirely anxious with no other feelings present. Usually when my worst times have occurred, I feel this way. I become Mr. Anxiety and Mr. Hypersensitivity.

Before knowing an alternative coping strategy, whenever I made a (perceived) mistake or had an uncomfortable experience, I mulled over, dwelled on, and recaptured all the antecedent factors that could have explained my behavior. I revisited what others' motivations may have been to act the way they did. I did these things while telling myself not to, though some of me thought that it was reasonable to discover why I had gotten so anxious. I felt as though I had to figure out why I felt the way I did and come to a resolution. I wanted to eliminate the bad feeling as quickly as possible. My overthinking sensitized me to the social environment. Of course, I was engaging in mental compulsions and overanalyzing. I was trying to reduce my anxiety. I knew this was not helpful. But, the pull of the moment compelled me to continue onward.

It was reasonable to ponder the causes and motivations of a social interaction, but I was doing it excessively. In my attempt to put the pieces back together again and feel whole, fine, and living in the present, I thought of and envisioned many things. I could not get a handle on all of it. I needed to see everything all at once and completely, but this apparently was impossible. If one piece did not quite fit, I might as well not have even tried to put the puzzle together. There was always at least one piece that did not meet the requirements. One or two that would not bend or fold to mold itself into the shape that I needed. Despite many desperate attempts to bring everything together, it would not work. Things did not feel right. I was resigned to the fact that I was going to have to think about it further.

I realize, upon scrutinizing the sequence of aforementioned events, the level of involvement of my reasoning and intellect. I'm a smart guy, but it does not matter what a person's IQ score is when emotions are involved. First, I'm running from the uncomfortable feeling, thinking that it does not make sense to feel this way. In fact, it does not matter if it makes sense or not; feel the emotion. Whether that emotion is anxiety, guilt, jealousy, or bitterness, feel the feeling. Don't automatically dismiss feelings. Yes, feelings are often misguided and are certainly not facts; however, they do provide useful information if we only pay attention.

My anxious and hypersensitive feelings frequently occur when other feelings become unbearable, intolerable, tiring, and burdensome. My OCD can act as a defense against other uncomfortable feelings. Obsessing and engaging in compulsions becomes one's primary manner of coping with discomfort. The problem with an obsessive-compulsive coping style is that the real reason that one feels uncomfortable gets distorted or blocked out, and an OCD coping style by its very definition and nature keeps the discomfort alive much longer than it needs to be.

As previously stated, sometimes I would get so wrapped up in OCD, and it was difficult to come up with techniques that would be useful to assist fighting the anxiety and hypersensitivity. For example, when I was a graduate student, I attended many meetings. There were staff psychiatrists, psychologists, and social workers in attendance most of the time. One particular day, we were to have a group meeting with some adolescent patients and some of the professional staff members. Everyone sat down, and then to the surprise of all, the director of the hospital came in. I had seen him a few times around the hospital grounds and had heard about his wealth, professional knowledge (he was a renowned psychiatrist himself), and influence at the hospital. He was a very important man.

When he walked in, I started thinking about where he was going to sit. Actually, that was what everyone was thinking. I felt very self-conscious, anxious, and sensitive. There were no extra chairs and a couple of people were already standing. I knew that as a student I was at the bottom of the pecking order. Yet, there were other students there, too. *Why should I be the one who gives up my chair?* I kept going back and forth, doing and undoing reasons to remain where I was or to stand and give him my chair. I was completely torn. I felt eyes staring at me, but my body would not move. I did not want to get up in front of twenty people. I hated being the center of attention. Consequently, I stayed put. He finally found a chair.

After the meeting, my supervisor talked to me about the uneasiness of knowing exactly what to do when this doctor entered the room and was looking for a comfortable place to relax and listen to the meeting. She had observed this sensitive situation before. She was aware that I felt anxious and told me that sometimes one just has to do things in spite of his or her discomfort and ambivalence. She believed that I should have given up my chair. I knew that I should have, too; she gave me permission to feel this way. It would have been better if I had given him my chair. I would not be feeling as anxious as I did.

I vowed that if I ever got stuck in an awkward, OCD-producing situation, I would go ahead and do the most helpful thing. I was not going to allow the presence of anxiety and OCD thinking from keeping me doing the appropriate thing. I knew how difficult it was to move when high levels of anxiety were present. But, I was not going to allow it to dictate what I did.

Ironically, the next day my assertiveness was tested. My client lived near Senator Strom Thurmond in a condo complex. She had told me this before. Well, I was walking through the lobby area after getting off the elevator after an in vivo session. To my surprise, the Senator was walking through the lobby all alone towards me. It was in the evening. I had heard that in the mornings there was practically an entire convoy that took him to work. I was surprised to see him all alone. Anyway, I was anxious in his presence. Nobody else was around and it was only the two of us there. I started to think of ways to avoid him or things to do that would make him leave me alone. I wanted, but didn't want to meet him or say "hi." A lifetime of OCD material whizzed through my mind in a flash. Memories of the "director of the hospital" incident were fresh in my mind. I knew that I wanted to face my anxiety. *What am I going to do in the presence of a famous person.* The next thing I knew, I was shaking hands with the famous, longstanding Senator and saying "hello." It's great when a plan comes together!

My recommendation to others who have OCD and/or sensitivities is to practice relaxation techniques (diaphragmatic breathing, visualization, deep muscle relaxation) and exercise on a daily basis to reduce the overall, everyday level of arousal that you experience. With frequent practice, you are better physiologically and emotionally equipped to manage greater levels of anxiety. Also, intentionally place yourself in difficult, anxiety-provoking situations (do not practice relaxation techniques right before, during, or soon after an exposure to an anxiety-inducing stimulus) as frequently as possible. It will be difficult as anything is at first, but with repetition, you will improve. Ultimately, your anxiety will not fuel the fire of more self-doubt, uncertainty, and apprehension.

Be aware of your vulnerabilities and get sufficient sleep. Live life to its fullest. Don't avoid situations because they are or may be uncomfortable. Be aware when you are jumping to conclusions about what "everyone" must be thinking when you don't have objective evidence that supports your belief.

Because of what I have learned over the years, now I am able to employ a more proactive, assertive style of coping that certainly helps with my anxiety and my hypersensitivities. I'm not just waiting around for bad things to happen and bad feelings to arrive. I am being active, taking initiative, and thinking ahead, because if I get stymied in OCD quicksand, it is very difficult to get out. The benefits of engaging in a more assertive style of managing uncomfortable feelings are many. One of the more important ones, and a benefit that I sometimes did not understand in the past, is the ability to expend energy on more than solely keeping the OCD going. I was so busy that I did not, or was unable to, think about strategies that I could employ the next time I ran into a similar situation. In a healthy way, another benefit is the reduction of anxiety.

In social situations, I was hypersensitive at times. OCD and hypersensitivity did not always coexist. For me, in many social situations, when the anxiety decreased, so did my hypersensitivities.

Chapter 8

SHAKEN, . . . SHAKEN *AND* STIRRED

I was just beginning my last year as a graduate student in social work. It was September, 1994 and I was a young adult. I had received my third choice for an internship site, but still felt fortunate to have it. The hospital was a very well known, highly reputed psychiatric facility. I wanted to be steeped in psychoanalytic thought since this perspective was the springboard for so much of mental health theory and practice today. Learning as much as I could at the hospital would prepare me for anything that would be thrown my way after school (or so I thought).

Not only was I a student at a hospital with a lofty reputation, intimidating colleagues, and high expectations, but my girlfriend Lynn and I were engaged to be married. I had asked her to marry me on her birthday. We spent much time and energy together for the many preparations for the wedding. We were very much in love and waiting in anticipation for the big day. Projecting myself into the future, I doubted my ability to do everything we were setting out to do. *Am I really going to get married? Will it work out?*

Besides being a graduate student and a future husband, I was also an employee. I wore many hats and played many roles; there were significant stressors in my life that made OCD more likely to surface. I worked at a residential treatment house for developmentally-disabled adolescents. Residents included wheelchair-bound people who required total care and individuals suffering from autism, mental retardation, and epilepsy due to head trauma. It was a very challenging job because of problematic behaviors like yelling, running away, hitting, kicking, threatening suicide, amongst others. Despite its intense demands, it was also very rewarding to be able to help teenagers live a more productive and fulfilling life. The relationships I forged with the residents were very special. However, there were behaviors from time to time that required the staff's special, undivided attention. The most difficult behavior problems that we faced occurred when an individual became very angry and started endangering his or her own safety, or the safety and well-being of others.

I frequently wondered and sometimes doubted if I had done enough or had acted in a proactive rather than a reactive way to prevent these angry outbursts. I had learned the importance of assertiveness at the hospital. At a minimum, I had to gain control of the situation once it started, and sometimes I obsessed about whether or not I had reacted in a proper and reasonable manner. Typically, my conclusion was that a "better course of action could have been taken." The greater the frequency, intensity, and duration of my obsessive thinking, the greater my level of uncertainty was regarding my professional competence. I knew it was a trap, but pulling myself out of it and not being seduced by the obsessions were very, very difficult. At times, it seemed impossible. My mind kept telling me that just one more thought, or one more thought deliberated about in another way would make all the difference. Of course, this was an illusion.

It is well-known that any one individual's behavior is not always predictable. Likewise, his or her behavior may not be immediately controllable. As an aspiring health care professional, I knew this. However, my OCD wanted, no, it needed for me to feel more in control of certain volatile situations. Like some OCD sufferers, I felt responsible for other peoples' feelings, thoughts, actions, and negative things that happened to them. I had a distorted perception of responsibility for other's undesirable behavior; I felt responsible for the consequences of others' acts. I did not believe that what I had done was correct, complete, and thorough. At times, I did not think that I did a good enough job. In fact, I felt as though I caused harm to them.

A prime example of the experience of feeling overresponsible for something I wasn't responsible for occurred at work. It was dinner time and three residents and one other staff member were eating spaghetti. I must have cooked it because pasta was the extent of my culinary expertise. The fourth resident was in her room, just sitting there looking lifeless. We tried to get her to join the rest of us, but she didn't respond. Now and then she would get into a dazed, confused state, particularly after experiencing a seizure. Therefore, the behavior she exhibited was nothing unusual.

In the meantime, I was helping a girl by cutting up her food so that she could eat it. I felt very good, and in that moment I was living in the present instead of living weeks, months, or years back in the past. But the present was bombarding me at an accelerated rate. OCD was right around the corner. I could sense it. How did I know this? It was the manner in which I began mentally warding off my anxiety. I repeatedly told myself that everything was OK, and that I was doing a good job performing my work duties. In addition, I kept saying that everything would turn out fine. I was even saying that it was OK that everything was OK. I wanted so badly for everything to be good and "right" inside my mind, neatly sorted and organized, and my feelings to be positive. In short, I was making myself very susceptible to OCD.

Meanwhile, a male resident had called me a "Meathead." I had to keep reminding myself that we often joked with each other and it never meant anything. I had to pay attention to what I was doing to ensure that the knife I was using to cut up the meat was not near my skin. I had to make sure of everything! I thought to myself, "I'm a little too close," then I would say, "That's ridiculous, no I'm not." These words continued to echo in my head. I wondered if I wanted to cut myself since I kept thinking about it. Obviously, my mind was not at peace. Repeatedly telling myself, "Go with the flow," and "Just experience the anxiety, go with it," became obsessive. I couldn't keep up with everything. *Can't everybody slow down and let me process what's going on in my life and at this table, both internally and externally?* The girl wanted her food cut up in smaller pieces, and another resident wanted something else.

Then, a female coworker called to me from the absent girl's room. She had gone to check on her and to see if we could get her to prepare herself for her parent's forthcoming arrival. She called me into the room to see if I could get a response out of her. Actually, I didn't know at the time why she had called me. I thought that maybe the female resident had suffered a seizure, and that my colleague needed help in maintaining her safety. So I dutifully went to see what was happening.

While trying to catch up to the mental chatter in my mind, attempting to "stay current" with other peoples' demands, needs, and responses, and my own cognitions, feelings, and overt behavior, I walked back to the room. In other words, I was ripe for the picking. There was just too much riding on what I or anyone else did. I had reached my OCD boiling point and could not do anything about it. However, I had to do my job. I had to go back there and see what was happening. I dreaded this walk because I realized what might happen. From time to time, the girl became agitated, and I did not want to deal with anything resembling agitation. Walking back through the hallway, turning the corner to go into her room, a lightning-fast thought came to me. I may have bumped up against the wall or her door with my foot. A strange sensation raced to my mind from my right foot. Trying to interpret the incoming data as quickly as possible before going into the room, I exhausted myself. Still not feeling right about whatever happened with my foot (later, after the intensity of the moment faded, I was able to say, "Who cares what happened to my foot, leg, arm, and the rest of my damn body!"), I entered the room.

I walked up to the girl and placed my hand on her back and asked her, "What's going on?" Bringing my worst fears to life, she became extremely hostile. She rose from her wheelchair and stood wobbling against the closet doors. She threw two objects and then made fists in an expression of intense anger. I had worked with this particular girl for over a year prior to this episode and had never observed her so out-of-control. I attempted to assist her, but she was in no state of mind to receive any help. She was strong enough to do some damage to someone or something. My female colleague was trying to keep herself safe; she was extremely frightened by this display of aggression and defiance. I tried to reach over to her, but I couldn't get to her. The resident continued yelling, punching, and kicking at me, and making it impossible for me to help her.

As you guessed, I was very anxious during this incident. Naturally, I did not want her or anyone else to get hurt, yet I felt helpless to successfully fulfill my duties as an employee. My anxiety continued to climb as the seconds ticked by. My body and mind froze as I realized the desperate, uncontrollable situation we were in. Everything started moving in slow motion as the hopelessness of the scene registered.

My OCD soars in times like this when I can't do what I need to do. Furthermore, my anxiety skyrockets even more when I feel that I may be held accountable for something bad happening to another person. Public accountability is terrible, but private, persistent personal feelings of failure torture a soul just as much, if not more.

I hate this, not being able to do what I have to and should do! I can feel the level of my anxiety and feelings of futility reach very dangerous heights. *Oh, no! She fell down! She fell down! I feel just awful! Did she hit her head against anything? What can I do? She fell! I cannot take that back. She's throwing clothes at me and not allowing me to help her. Just let her get this out of her system. She can't stay this angry for very long. Her parents will be here soon anyways. Oh, no! They are going to be mad at me because she will not be ready to leave. I can't believe this! She is throwing the clothes that she was taking home. They are scattered all over the room. Should I just let her play her rage out? . . . or, should I try to see if she injured herself in the fall? Isn't that what a good employee would do? But she won't let me.* Heights of anxiety were present that have been associated with longstanding obsessions in the past, even obsessions that have endured for years. I would have done anything to have gotten out of there, but I couldn't. I was stuck in that room trying to do something that was impossible, or at least seemed to be impossible. *But it shouldn't be impossible. I must be messing up terribly. It must be the OCD that is keeping me from saving this woman. I should be able to help her. Other people here could help her.* The OCD preoccupied me and made it difficult to move and initiate action. Finally, she sat down on her bed and stopped throwing anything. *Oh God, she fell off of the bed! If only I had been closer to her, this wouldn't have happened. I allowed her to have another chance at hurting herself. I can't believe I allowed her to fall off her bed! This whole thing is my fault!*

The worst consequence of this incident was that I could not do anything to undo it. I could not engage in any kind of compulsion to eliminate or reduce my anxiety. Imaginably revisiting the event only served to dredge up more questions and to further erode my self-esteem. I wished that I was a handwasher at that moment so that all I had to do was to wash my hands and my absolute, total nervousness would be brought down to a manageable, tolerable level. Any other symptom would be better than this big permanent black mark on my psychic record that would never be erased.

Every person suffering from OCD wishes, at one point or another, that they "only had to put up with something else." They think anything else can't be as bad as what they are experiencing now. Certainly, it seems that way. But, in reality, no symptom manifestation is inherently less painful than any other. Handwashers, checkers, counters, and others, can, and do experience the same extremely high levels of anxiety. When one is going through a very difficult time, anything looks better at that moment than the present problem. Moreover, the more one engages in any particular ritual, the harder it is to break away from it. Whether speaking about washing, checking, or mental ritualizing, this principle is true.

It was clear that I felt overresponsible for the welfare of the girl. At the time, my anxiety was so high that I had a distorted view of my role in protecting the resident. It took me two years to be emotionally comfortable about this event. I obsessed about the whole incident, dissecting each instant and analyzing my behavior. I spent countless hours ritualizing by recounting and revisiting the entire scene. Later, I ascertained that I was not responsible for her actions. (Paradoxically, the amount of time spent trying to resolve my unpleasant and intrusive thoughts and feelings is directly proportional to the pain that I suffered. In brief, the more I ritualized, the more it set me back.

Frequently, I am able to quickly work through things in my mind, logically sifting through all nagging internal experiences, and make sense of it all. Hopefully, after doing this, I feel better. However, I knew that this situation was different. It had a different feel to it. I could not make everything OK in my mind regardless of whether it was in real life or not. I felt awful no matter what I did, and this feeling was not abating as usual. I knew that it would take a long time to emotionally process this psychic scar.

The girl's parents arrived fifteen minutes after the violent outburst. It was their custom to see the girl every month. We were expecting them, and upon entering their daughter's bedroom, they witnessed the chaotic effects of her volatile behavior. They advised me not to feel bad about what had happened because it was not my fault. They had observed numerous angry outbursts over the years and understood and accepted them on some level. I thought that their intentions to put me at ease were good, but that it was too late to do anything about my most recent obsession. My obsession was like my phone number listed on a telemarketer's list; there was no way to remove it.

After the angry resident and her parents left the home, I excused myself, went into the bathroom to gather my thoughts, and tried to make some sense out of what had just transpired. I was in an all-encompassing fog cognitively and emotionally and had a very difficult time trying to think rationally about the incident. I was not psychotic; I knew what was happening and what had really occurred. I had no delusions or hallucinations, but I had a terrible time trying to cope with the level of anxiety that I had just started experiencing. It seemed to me that since my anxiety was extremely high, I must have really screwed up. I thought that there must be a direct relationship between my level of anxiety and the magnitude of my error. (Of course, this is an unhealthy, irrational way of thinking. Emotional reasoning is what professionals call the act of utilizing only your feelings to come to a conclusion or solution about something.)

I was taking deep breaths in the bathroom and attempting to bring some semblance of peace back, but I knew that I had crossed the line in the obsessional sand. The enormous level of anxiety I felt, and the resulting doubts and insecurities about my competence to do a good job were going to endure for a long time. I knew this through experience, because when I had crossed a certain elevated level of anxiety in a situation as emotionally threatening to me as this one was in the past, I had experienced long-lasting OCD. I wanted to cry, but I couldn't. I wanted to think rationally about what had just happened, but I couldn't.

I felt completely defeated and emotionally blank. I was numb and did not want to feel, for if I did I would risk feeling more pain and anxiety. At that moment, I did not want to feel anything. I felt very uncomfortable, anxious, and guilty, and I defended against all of them. For three days, I did not think too much about that night and the angry girl, choosing to suppress everything about them. I went back to a staff meeting on the fourth day, and the subject of the episode came up. I did not want anything to do with the episode, however, being an employee, I was forced to listen and participate in the discussion.

The topic of the resident's safety was a recurring one. I needed my supervisor to tell me in no uncertain terms that there was nothing more that I could have done, and that the girl did get angry from time to time no matter what you did. Without regard to my inner voice screaming for mercy, the supervisor, after acknowledging the fact that the girl was very difficult to handle at times, wondered aloud if anything more could have been done to avert the incident. He surmised that maybe someone could have prevented this woman from falling if someone had helped her keep her balance. He believed that if this had been done, the entire scene would not have played out like it did. The staff would have had more control and reached her before she fell down. I was horrified that more possibilities were being explored. I knew that it was healthy and reasonable to discuss different options about what to do in challenging situations. Nonetheless, my anxiety mounted, and I felt as if I had to defend myself against an onslaught of things I could or should have done. I did not say much at the meeting, except to make the staff aware of the struggle that took place to maintain the resident's safety.

It is healthy to confront anxiety by talking it out, even if that means, no, especially if that means that your level of anxiety increases as you talk. Let yourself go with the flow of the anxiety. It takes practice. At first, it feels almost masochistic to engage in activities or put yourself in a position where your anxiety increases. You are inducing anxiety for a reason. Your goal is to become desensitized (or habituated), or get used to, the anxiety you feel about a particular event or stimulus. You are not just getting anxious with no ultimate goal in mind. A person's body adjusts to the temperature of water when he or she enters a pool, and your nervous system will do the same with anxiety, desensitizing itself to the new realities of more frequent, intense, and longer-lasting anxieties.

Over time, my obsession and concurrent anxiety diminished in intensity and personal meaning for me. Why? Well, time helps to a certain extent. Attaining some emotional distance from the event by viewing it through different colored lenses helped reduce my anxiety as well. More importantly, I continued to work at the group home. Believe me, I had many thoughts about quitting and finding another job. Nevertheless, I realized that life was going to throw me these curve balls and that I needed to learn how to improve my batting average. My perseverance ensured that I would finally let go and get through the emotional quicksand.

It is very important to manage and tolerate the anxiety you are experiencing. It is self-defeating and unrealistic to have as a goal that you are going to eliminate or get rid of the discomfort completely. In deed, by attempting to rid yourself of anxiety, you are playing into the OCD's hand. There will be an illusion before you of attaining complete and utter tranquility with your OCD symptoms. You begin thinking, "If I only do this . . . if I only did that . . . then all would be well." That is precisely how OCD depresses, shames, and erodes an individual's self-esteem. Paradoxically, by allowing the obsession or fear to enter, hang-out, and be present, you can gain more peace than by trying to cleanse yourself of discomfort. Anxiety and stress are necessary components of every human. They serve to protect and defend each individual. Hence, erasing anxiety and stress from an emotional landscape is impossible and dangerous to your existence. Each person must make the decision to live realistically and reasonably with his or her OCD.

I am not any better or any different than anyone else suffering from OCD. If I can persevere, enjoy life, and continue to grow, I am confident that my fellow sufferers can do the same. As many people with OCD, when I got through the "angry girl" incident, emotionally integrating and processing its impact, a vacuum appeared. All of a sudden, there was this space in my head that I did not know what to do with. I wasn't anxious any more. Keeping busy helps to fill in that gap; however, this does not always suffice. Sometimes sufferers become nervous about not being anxious.

The last thing that you want to have happen, right after you endure two years worth of pain and suffering, is for something else to upset the balance. In the past, I have made the mistake of trying to protect myself from myself. I would not participate in an activity because I ran the risk of "picking up" another obsession to replace the one that I had just overcome. I found that the more I protected myself, the more I was hurting myself. And no one picks up an obsession like they do a virus. OCD sufferers need to continue to participate in life. For if you don't, the OCD wins and you lose. Losing is not an option.

I recall feeling great and relieved about surviving the long bout with my "angry girl" obsession and the anxiety generated by it. My mind was racing wildly again, trying to keep up with everything. This experience was akin to what I went through before the entire "angry woman" obsession. It seemed as though my mind was searching for something to latch onto. If I could only find something to obsess about, this would stop the madness of attempting to keep up with my thoughts. Keeping up was an impossible task; I tried participating in life, not avoiding any activities as I had done before, and absorbing myself in my surroundings. I also used deep breathing techniques to relax. Obsessing about an event for a long time was obviously a very unpleasant possibility; it had occurred in the past. It appeared as though I had nowhere else to go. I was caught in a double bind and would lose either way I looked at it. If I fell behind my OCD, I was preoccupied. And if I continued to exert much energy to catch up to my thoughts, I was running in my hamster wheel, exhausted and spent (for no good reason). It appeared that my mind was conspiring against me and I seemed incapable of stopping it.

New thoughts rampaged through my mind about the "angry woman" incident; I still did not feel thoroughly at peace with myself about it. I began thinking that maybe I could have handled the entire situation differently. *Maybe I could have avoided a lot of pain and suffering. What if I had acted differently that night? What if I had only helped myself, befriended myself? My life may be totally different now. If only I had exposed myself to the source of my anxiety, and prevented a compulsive response, I would have been much better off.*

Since E/RP therapy was a therapeutic modality that I was a little familiar with and learning more about, I began to take my newfound knowledge and ask myself questions about the past. They were questions that I had no business going back over, but questions that seemed very natural to ask. *What if I had done E/RP therapy from the start? Could I have reduced the total amount of agony and wasted energy I used for my obsessions and compulsions? Should I have known about how to handle certain situations better?* But, I did. I kept working at the house. I did not add the fuel of avoidance to the OCD fire. My therapist concurred that, given the circumstances, I had behaved in a courageous manner, standing up to my anxiety. But I wasn't so certain about whether or not I had avoided the girl's bedroom at times because of anxiety.

It was evident that there was some exposure to the source of my anxiety; I continued to work at the residency for another nine months after the incident. My responsibilities included continuing to work with the "angry girl." Due to the greater comfort level of employees working in bathrooms with residents of the same sex, time working with this girl could diminish if a female staff member was present. Avoidance for its own sake wasn't what I desired (most of the time), just an occasional break away from her. In their calm, happy moments, the residents were fun to work with. *I know there was some exposure, but was it the right kind? Was it like the E/RP I read a few pages about?*

It didn't matter! It was another mystery, an additional puzzle that had to be solved or resolved. It had happened in the past, so what if the procedures for E/RP were not followed precisely? *What do you mean "so what?" Maybe not acting in the "perfect" way would leave scars. Maybe I had not educated myself enough about E/RP?* I've always been afraid that one of my obsessions was going to lead to a permanent, dysfunctional, even a dependent condition. And the anxiety that I experienced about the "angry girl" was still very high. In sum, I didn't want to go nuts.

A week after the "angry girl incident," I spoke to a friend who also suffered from OCD. He recommended that I keep in mind that this was what happened to me when OCD struck. He said that I should acknowledge that my level of anxiety was very, very high, and that it would not remain at this very high level for much longer. By recognizing the entire thought process as part and parcel of the disorder, I would be better able to expedite the process of letting go of the obsessions, feel more connected with the life that I was living, and go on with the rest of my life.

My friend tried to help, but talking to him evoked greater levels of anxiety, self-doubt, and anger because everything that he suggested had not been done. I knew that in these very high anxiety situations, that nipping it in the bud and getting a grip on things early was very important. Precious time had already slipped by, and it must be too late to try to relive what had already taken place a week before. *If only I had acted sooner, immediately after my anxiety rose. Then, nothing would be wrong with me.* Everything that I did to help myself increased my anxiety even more. Talking to a friend, going to therapy, and going to work could not help me escape the tormenting cascade of interminable thoughts and questions in my mind.

My psychiatrist at the time wanted to experiment with some different medications to see if the degree, frequency, and duration of my symptoms could improve. He had an interesting theory. My description of my internal experiences about the "angry girl" led him to think of my obsessing as maybe being the result of a traumatic event. Perhaps a medication that treated Post-Traumatic Stress Disorder (PTSD) would be efficacious. The doctor stated that part of the clinical picture of PTSD commonly included a rehashing of old material. *Well, hey, that's me! Maybe I have PTSD. No, I can't have what rape victims and soldiers sometimes are afflicted with! Things can get unbearable from time to time, but I can't have that, too.* In PTSD, the nervous system is stressed to the point that all incoming sensory, emotional, and cognitive information cannot be integrated as it usually is. Thoughts and feelings become all jumbled up and aren't experienced normally. Why is this? Because the situation and the environmental stimuli are not typical and common. For example, some Viet Nam veterans are diagnosed with PTSD. Were their surroundings commonplace? No, of course not.

Although I was not in a life or death, let the bullets fly sort of experience, it was not a typical situation. The woman did not usually act the way that she displayed that evening. Even when she got angry, in most instances she did not punch, kick, bite, and fall to the ground. My nervous system **perceived** the experience as a threat, and according to the doctor's theory, a perception was all that was needed. Maybe I now suffered from PTSD or a variant. I have always tried any medication recommended by my psychiatrist and have done whatever it took to help myself. I believe that God helps those who help themselves. So I tried Depakote. It didn't work; it made me very sedated. But I would not have known that it did not work if I hadn't tried it.

Approximately a month after the incident, I watched a videotape concerning the treatment of OCD. During the viewing, the doctor said that it was important to address an OCD symptom immediately, or at least soon after its appearance. (This is not the case. It is <u>more</u> beneficial to manage a symptom earlier.) Misinterpreting the content of the tape made me feel even more inconsolable and hopeless. I felt as though I had really, really screwed up and that I would obsess about the incident for the rest of my life. Since the incident had already occurred, I could not do anything about it, so I had to suffer. My conclusion is laughable and absurd now as I write, but during the dark days, I assure you, it wasn't.

Later, I realized that there was something that could be done, despite the "tardiness" of the intervention. I couldn't undo what had been done, but I could <u>react </u>differently. I could expose myself to the anxiety of the event and then prevent my typical compulsive, ruminative response. The most effective way of managing a fear is to confront and attack it. Toward that end, I created a three-minute endless-loop audiotape (similar to an answering machine tape that is available at electronics stores) using my own voice to describe the events that prompted my incompetent feelings. For example, picturing the resident falling down was my most frightening memory. Therefore, I recorded on the tape, "The resident wobbled and fell down while I could only stand and watch. I did nothing. He may have injured himself. I may be incompetent for allowing him to fall to the ground." I listened to the tape every day for two weeks. Creating endless-loop audiotapes is an effective E/RP technique. I addressed my uncertainty about my job performance by using the words may, might, and maybe. I exposed myself to uncertainty; that's what I needed to do.

I needed to be more comfortable with being uncomfortable, with not knowing everything or each aspect of something. I knew that I performed well at my job, but the doubt and the emotional distress that I experienced about whether it was "good enough" was at the root of the obsession. In my case, it was necessary to use these words that connoted uncertainty to raise my anxiety.

Certainly, my anxiety rose as I listened to the details on the tape, especially when   I labeled myself "incompetent." It was very uncomfortable and anxiety-provoking to listen to the tape. At any rate, the real events, memories, and obsessions triggered therefrom were already bothering me, so what did I have to lose by listening? The words inadequate and unprofessional rang in my head over and over again because the word incompetent reminded me of them. I listened to the tape until my anxiety decreased by more than one-half of its peak measure. You always follow the one-half rule: you need to wait until your anxiety decreases by at least fifty percent when performing an exposure. More is even better.

What were the results of such a crazy sounding audiotape scheme? The entire incident became boring, and the absurdity, ridiculousness, and excessiveness of the entire obsession became more evident than ever. I became "biologically bored" with the material by repeatedly practicing it. Even if I had been incompetent, it was not productive to obsess and mull over the same thing time and time again.

You might be thinking, "He's not just obsessive, but a little masochistic as well." You might be thinking that this sounds like a lot of difficult work. Well, you're right (not about masochism, though). To sit there and become anxious listening to the tape was enough to make me want to rush over and break the tape player by smashing it against the wall. It sent chills down my spine, made my stomach twist into knots, and my head seemed to get heavier. Nevertheless, the results were normally positive.

I can go on and on and sound like a cheerleader, exhorting you to perform daily, direct (e.g. keep touching something contaminated, continue listening to the tape, etc.), and prolonged exposures. Having a therapist guide, direct, and coach encourages you and aids immensely. The difference between people getting better or not improving often has to do with their level of motivation and the amount of practicing they do on their own. People need practice and repetition to break out of old, unhealthy behavior and thinking patterns, and to establish new ones. There are no shortcuts, although it does not have to take but a few weeks of work to change your life. What will it be?

Chapter 9

WEDDING DAY

Lynn is a wonderful woman, overflowing with compassion and love. She is a registered nurse who works in an intensive-care unit. Her caring for others is evident in many other spheres of her life. I knew that she was right for me after only a few months together. We had started dating in September of 1989 and got engaged on her birthday, in March of 1994. We had spent a lot of time together and really got to know each other. However, being engaged (and not just dating) involves a completely new set of expectations, a new identity, and a new role. Wedding plans were in the works, and we were being introduced to others as a future couple. Everyone said, "They're engaged" whenever we met someone new, including our numerous trips to check on various reception sites, photographers, cake bakers, etc.

When Lynn and I met each other in 1989, it was in mental health hospital. No, it's not what you think! We both worked there. I was a psychiatric technician and she was a student nurse extern there. I called her after noticing her at a work party. She was very attractive and appeared almost angelic to me; she seemed so sweet and innocent. We started dating on September 22. Therefore, we dated six years before we got married.

In 1994, it was her birthday and I had been seriously considering asking her to marry me for a few months. I did not know what I was waiting for other than wanting there to be no doubt or worries present. Being a biologist, my father told me that her "biological clock was ticking." I assured myself that no one got married being one hundred percent certain of what the future held. I believed that she was good for me and that she was the right one, but the more I questioned myself and the more time elapsed, I felt less certain about a decision. I kept going back and forth, back and forth in my mind as I drove to a local supermarket. I was playing "OCD pong" in my mind as my heart raced and my head began to hurt. The bright, sunny day seemed to signal that a higher power approved of this life-long relationship commitment. Finally, I decided to take the bull by the horns and make a decision. Yes, I would marry her! I made up my mind at the supermarket to ask her when I arrived at her apartment. The timing seemed right and it was her birthday. This would make a great birthday gift for her.

I returned to her apartment and sat down next to her. We were talking about her birthday when I popped the question. Despite waiting for me to ask her for so long, she told me later that she was surprised that I had asked her then, but she managed to say "yes." I felt calmer since I knew that I felt good about the decision. After I gave myself a definitive answer and she gave me an affirmative response, the pressure seemed to wane.

As the months sped by, I was feeling even better about getting married. The engagement had reduced my anxiety; it allowed me to practice an intermediary role between single and married. Lynn and I, with her mother's help, planned the entire wedding. The day was rapidly approaching.

The night before the wedding, I was out with the boys at a bar having a few drinks. I had a few too many, but luckily was not hung over the next day. Sometimes I told myself that I was just going to have a good time, and if obsessions came, so be it. They were not going to stop me from enjoying myself. By this point, I had learned to make more of an effort to enjoy myself when the obsessions came.

On the day of the wedding, I woke up late at my parent's house. The wedding was on Saturday at 4 P.M., so there was plenty of time to get ready. I was excited, calm, and cool. When I knew it was safe to go to her apartment because Lynn would not be there, I went to pick up my tuxedo and clothes. She wasn't there and I was not much later than I had anticipated. There was only one thing that I had to do before I could go to my parent's house in peace.

To make sure that nobody was going to rob her place while we were gone, I wanted to ask someone to watch the apartment. We were worried because Lynn had unwittingly sent money to someone who was pretending to be a social security representative. We found out later, after she sent the money, that fraud was involved. Our wedding date was on the form she had sent in and we were suspicious that the culprits may try to break into our apartment, realizing that many gifts would be there already. Bad people would also know that we might be out of town for a while on our honeymoon. No one was home next door to ask such a favor. I saw someone outside at the swimming pool and thought that it was another neighbor. I hopped into my car and figured that on my way to my parent's house I would ask him. Well, I got out of the car, approached the pool, and called the man over. As he came over to me, I realized that this was not my neighbor, but only a guy who resembled him. I told him that I had the wrong person, turned around, and walked quickly back to my car. I was very embarrassed and anxious about committing such an egregious error. I perceived it as a terrible mistake due to my perfectionism and hypersensitivity, but the man surely shrugged it off quickly. All kinds of thoughts were swirling around in my mind. They were all incomplete thoughts and ideas, nothing that I could get a good handle on.

My thoughts probably went something like this: *How could I have done that? Who was that? House robbed! Embarrassing, no, it's no, yes it is. House*

robbed! My God, two hours until the wedding and I'm a mess! I can't go through with it. Fool of myself. House robbed! He thinks I'm gay. What? House robbed? No, I'm not gay. I'm getting married!"
       I started to shake on the way to my parents. I had a hard time keeping the car pointing straight and in my lane. *I'm not going to think about this gay thing. I only asked him a question, that is all. He doesn't think I'm gay because I thought he was another person.* My hands and arms were telling me that something unpleasant or even dangerous could be ahead. I remembered my therapist telling me that many individuals with OCD performed quite well in real-life anxiety-generating situations. They are accustomed to feeling anxiety and know instinctively and intuitively how to cope with it. They feel more comfortable feeling uncomfortable. Something else that helped me cope was to recall that we had had a rehearsal and there was really nothing that I could mess up. "I do" were only two words.
       When I arrived at my parent's house, they reported that I appeared pale. My anxiety rose as the time to the beginning of the wedding neared. Typically, I didn't experience many physiological symptoms when I was anxious. When there were several, I knew that I was very anxious. On the way to the church, I was sweating some, my heart was beating very rapidly, and my head, arms and hands were shaking. My head was ready to explode with thoughts. I was a mess and wanted to melt into a puddle of water. I wanted to escape the insidious and throbbing anxiety. Trust in my therapist was waning because I was not so sure I would get through the wedding.
       However, to my surprise, when I arrived at the church an hour before the wedding, I felt relatively calm. There were things to do: finishing getting dressed; shaving; taking pictures; exchanging joyful sentiments; hugging relatives; and getting last-second instructions from the minister. Although I was still thinking about the incident at the pool two hours earlier, and all the exaggerated, out of proportion ramifications of my behavior, and of not finding someone to keep an eye on the apartment, I felt all right. *Shut up and pay attention. My goodness, I am going to get married to the woman that I love! What else can a man ask for?*
       In the minister's study minutes before the wedding, I began to worry about my tuxedo. Fears of not having my tails on my tuxedo just right burdened me. I did not want the embarrassment of wearing clothes that were not on correctly. I knew that I was extremely anxious because I started obsessing about old OCD themes. OCD fears of making a big mistake and not being sexually appropriate (dressed correctly, all covered up) nagged at me. Exposures were beneficial in therapy, but I was worried about different kind of "exposure." Each time that I sat down to try to relax, I thought about the tails on my tux and experienced more an more anxiety. My anxiety increased because I had never worn tails on a tuxedo before, and I did not know what to do with them when I sat down. I remember talking to my best man (my brother), and the minister, and distracting myself from the familiar OCD thoughts. Immediately before walking out to greet my beautiful bride, I took a few deep breaths and reminded

myself again that one form my OCD took when I was extremely anxious was to obsess about whether I was revealing too much and being sexually inappropriate. *This is just OCD. Don't worry about it! I would know if my pants were down. But maybe I would not know. Oh, come on, I'm not aware of everything, but I would not miss this important piece of information. Wait a minute, there must be one hundred people out there waiting for my entrance, and they will be watching me the whole ceremony. Don't sweat it John, it is solely the OCD.* Identifying and acknowledging the presence of OCD helped me to cope with my anxiety.

By the time we walked out in front of everyone, I was very anxious, but no particular obsession was front and center in my mind. At that point, I was probably too exhausted to expend energy obsessing. I could do nothing about the apartment when all the wedding festivities were happening, therefore it would serve no positive purpose to obsess and to detract from the here-and-now experiences. The rest was history, and of course, in spite of my worries, everything turned out wonderfully. The reception was a blur, four hours transformed into fifteen minutes. The apartment remained free of intruders throughout the day, reminding me that the vast majority of things we worry or obsess about never come to pass. Thus, I learned that it is best to concern myself only with controllable things.

PART II:
YEARS AS A THERAPIST

Chapter 10

PREGNANCY

I started working as a psychotherapist in the same year that I got married, 1995. My wife and I bought our first house together one year later, and were very happy together. In 1997, we had been thinking about having children sometime in the future, but the future was upon us. Lynn was three months pregnant and her stomach was beginning to protrude. It was a very exciting time for both of us, and we felt ready for what was to come in six months.

OCD symptoms often exacerbate in response to perceived or real negative or positive circumstances and feelings. Frustratingly, symptoms often develop around an issue or event that is very significant and meaningful. I remember an individual I once met who experienced debilitating symptoms after his wife gave birth. Powerful feelings of anxiety overwhelmed him. It is not unusual for any individual to doubt his or her parental capacities and abilities, particularly with his or her first kids. Add this useful, adaptive doubt to the ever-present feelings of doubt and uncertainty already percolating in the thoughts and feelings of individuals with OCD, and you can see how sufferers' lives are very difficult.

I mention all of the above as an introduction. Given my propensity to have anxious thoughts and feelings about the welfare of others that I am (or feel) responsible for, it seems almost predetermined that I would obsess about my wife's pregnancy in some manner. It hit close to home and a lot of emotion was tied up in seeing our child develop, hopefully in a healthy and happy manner. My perfectionism wanted the pregnancy to happen seamlessly, without any complications.

The very first time that I obsessed about a pregnancy-related situation occurred as soon as it possibly could have. When I found out that my wife was pregnant, I immediately began to wonder whether my thoughts at the exact time of conception focused exclusively on my love for her. For some reason, I felt compelled to revisit the time of conception and try to remember what was precisely on my mind. Questions zoomed in and out of my mind. I was mental ritualizing by analyzing and revisiting the scene to try to reduce my anxiety. I yelled at myself internally, telling myself to stop this nonsense. However, the strength of the fear overwhelmed my ability to cope well; it was very difficult stopping the questions. *Was my mind wandering then? I don't think so, it usually doesn't, but I can't remember for sure. Was I thinking about work? How about the activities that had transpired during the day? Did another woman enter my consciousness? Or maybe the mosquito bite on my right leg broke my concentration? What if the image or thought of another woman entered my mind at the "wrong" time? What would happen to the baby?*

In my thoughts, not only was the content of my cognitions important at the precise moment of conception, but also the actual day that conception occurred. Of course, it was difficult to always know the exact date of conception. So I tried to memorize every time my wife and I made love during a one to two week period and review every detail I could remember. Of course, this was an impossible task. The more I reviewed my memories, the worse the OCD became. Questions just led to more questions. I got anxious when our conversation turned to the topic of the conception date and the expected date of delivery. I found myself hoping that we conceived on certain dates and not others. I could remember some days better than others.

To combat my fears, I asked myself, "So what?" whenever I began to wonder about the consequences of conceiving at the "wrong" time. Responding to "What if . . .?" questions in this manner put the entire situation into perspective. *So what if I was thinking about something else at the exact moment of conception? So what if I didn't remember the precise date of conception? Was all this information really that important anyways? No, it wasn't.*

As previously stated, OCD often attaches itself to very meaningful life choices and events. Humans tend to search for meaning and purpose in thoughts and actions, thus it is only natural that uncomfortable, out-of-place, and untimely thoughts and images may appear to signify more than they really do. We frequently believe that there is a clear, discernible connection between our thoughts and the meaning derived from those thoughts. We are often fooled by OCD; anxiety can distort the meaning of thoughts and images. Even if I had another thought or image at conception, it didn't mean anything. We must get past the old, outdated Freudian notion that a thought means something else.

Later in the pregnancy, a few things occurred that helped to illustrate what the nature of my "baby" OCD was, how I responded to it, and how I tried to assist myself in managing the anxiety and uneasiness associated with developments in the pregnancy. The first instance happened in the morning when my wife and I were preparing to go to the doctor's office. The day marked that it was six days past our baby's due date and we were going to assure everyone, including ourselves, that the baby was in no distress and still thriving. The baby wanted to remain in its nice, warm confines; it was not ready to come out yet. I was very anxious about the baby's hesitancy to surface, and my anxiety triggered more anxiety at that moment. I went to the den to pick up my wallet and car keys. As usual, I quickly and adaptively checked to see that everything required for the trip was in my pockets or my hands. While mentally checking with myself, I walked over to the bathroom. All I had to do was brush my teeth and hair. (You know, a person with OCD must appear impeccably dressed and well groomed. No, not necessarily!) I moved to turn the light on in the bathroom. *Ooops! It was already on.* Right then and there I felt compelled to say something to myself along the lines of, "I went to turn the light on but it was already on. I didn't realize that it was on so that's why I performed those extra, unproductive movements." This time I did ritualize by saying this to myself and it did make me feel better. Something didn't sit well with me after goofing up and making the false movement toward the light switch. *I should have known better to make a mistake, no matter how small and trivial!*

Afterwards, I knew that the ritual was unnecessary to think. It meant that OCD got me and it hit smack in the middle of perfectionistic behavior. During the two or three minutes I spent in the bathroom, I began to think about what had just transpired. Most people did not feel compelled to think certain thoughts under the same circumstances. I tended to be more comfortable with explaining every little twitch and blink instead of allowing what had just happened to simply happen. I was very uncomfortable with "making mistakes," even if they were not really mistakes. I simply tried to turn a light on that was already on. *Shame on me!*

Here is another example of my anxiety emerging because of the pregnancy. It is also another insightful example of my tendency to combine my perfectionism with anxiety. As I said before, my perfectionism and anxiety had increased during the course of the pregnancy. My wife was in the bathroom checking her blood sugar, and I was sitting calmly and patiently alone in the examining room. The nurse practitioner walked in and said that she would need to use the fetal monitor that was lying beside me to see the baby in utero. She continued to come towards me and as I was trying to get out of her way, she brushed up against me. My hands and arms touched her somewhere. Touching someone or wondering whether I touched someone generated anxiety. Perhaps I had acted in an inappropriate sexual manner. *Perhaps she will think I'm a pervert or sexual deviant. What if I accidentally touched her breasts or bottom? I should not have been over there to begin with. I knew that the fetal monitor was going to be used today, but I still parked myself right next to it. I could have avoided this whole thing if I had only thought ahead of time and sat somewhere else. Wait a minute. I'm not going to obsess about this incident.* The chatter in my head continued to argue the two opposing sides of who was to blame. *First of all, that's the chair that I usually sit in. We're creatures of habit, right? I was tired anyway, I can't always think of these things ahead of time. No, that has nothing to do with it. I sat in that chair. So what? Anybody else may have, too. I didn't do anything wrong.*

Rationality started to assert itself. *Most importantly, there is nothing to worry about with this woman. I wish she would not have come over so quickly and had at least given me a chance to get out of the way. The examining table had left me no room to move. The only way to get out of her way was going towards her.* I felt trapped and there was no way out. That's why my anxiety escalated so quickly. I had no control over what the woman did. *Well, that's life. I don't like it because my anxiety skyrockets. People sometimes brush up against each other; cities would not exist if that was not permitted and expected. Don't worry about things you can't control; save your worry for the things you have some control over. But, I could have not sat . . . I don't want to hear it. At any rate, I'm sure she doesn't even remember it. I'm obsessing about it and she dropped the issue before picking it up.*

My perfectionism and anxiety continued to increase as the delivery date neared. I wanted a "perfect" child and I needed to challenge my OCD through rational responses, exposures, and by refraining from avoidance and rituals. I used the exposure of telling myself that the child was going to be imperfect and that there was nothing I could do about it. I never let my last thought be about a "perfect" child. I wanted to be a healthy, confident father, able to raise a healthy, confident child. I knew that I couldn't have a "perfect" child, and I also knew rationally that I didn't cause any bad things to happen to the child. Laughing at myself and thinking as rationally as possible also helped me to take some difficult steps during the pregnancy. I made it to the birth (relatively) unscathed. But, I wondered if I would keep obsessing about my role and responsibility in the welfare of my child in the future.

Chapter 11

DELIVERY AND BEYOND

How about that! I was a father! I made it through the entire pregnancy; I learned that they allowed someone with OCD to become a father. No, just kidding. This chapter will examine the births of both of my children and how my OCD and I reacted to them.

Lynn was admitted into the hospital at 6:30 P.M. on a Tuesday evening, and our daughter was born on Thursday morning at 7:04 A.M. Lynn and I had started quite a journey on Tuesday night. We did not get much sleep (especially Lynn) and we were getting frustrated that our baby was not cooperating. We wanted so much to finally touch, hold, and love our little baby.

My frustration and anxiety diminished upon seeing the confident expectation of a successful outcome on the faces of the professionals attending to my wife. The calmness present in the room served to keep me relatively tranquil and certain that everything was going as planned. By their actions, they reassured me that everything was under control. Tranquility and confidence surrounded me, and I made more of an effort to pay attention to it. It was important to observe how competent, experienced professionals behaved and try to think and act in a manner that reflected their grace under pressure. The doctors and nurses had delivered thousands of babies and the technology and understanding of the process was better than ever. Getting outside myself by observing self-assured, competent individuals function was an adaptive way of viewing events in a non-anxious light.

Lynn and I had attended Lamaze classes and had read a good deal about the birthing process. We had been encouraged to construct a birthing plan that would assist our doctors and ourselves with answers to questions about issues such as: epidural vs. no epidural, painkillers vs. no painkillers, circumcision vs. no circumcision, episiotomy vs. no episiotomy, etc. Well, the class was informative, interesting, and supportive; however, we could not apply much of the instructor's teaching because the baby was almost two weeks overdue. The amount of amniotic fluid surrounding the baby was low. There was no crisis, but there was some concern on the part of the doctor regarding the positioning of the baby and the baby's heart rate. Our doctor decided to induce labor. In class, we had focused almost exclusively on labor beginning at home, and most importantly, without the use of any drugs. The instructor was militant on this point, hammering away at her position each and every class. The class had unwittingly raised my anxiety because I was more aware of the irregularities of our situation.

Lynn and I had to adapt to our particular new set of circumstances. Lynn's contractions, despite tremendous effort, stamina, and breathing exercises, were very forceful and painful, and did not produce results at first. She required a painkiller and later an epidural. Our birthing plan seemed to fly out the window; our birthing experience did not reflect the type we had discussed in class. The piece of paper with the plan quietly and unobtrusively lay on a shelf at the side of the room. I noticed it but realized that it was essentially useless. *Maybe all of our wishes are not being met. Do the doctors know what course of action we ideally would like to follow?*

Finally, after we spent much of the night monitoring the baby's heart rate, the time came for the baby to be born. Lynn's legs were numbed and not under her control so I helped lift one leg up to aid her in pushing, while a nurse held up the other. I could not believe my eyes; the top of the baby's head was in sight. "Go Lynn, the baby is coming, you're doing a great job!" The entire thing was a miracle, one of those experiences that was so incredible and mysterious that it made you think that there really must be a Divine Presence somewhere, and it was right there in the hospital room.

The baby made her long-awaited arrival. I was worrying that maybe when the nurse told me to place Lynn's leg back on the support beam that it meant that I had done something wrong. I thought that the very fact that she had to say something meant that I had committed an error. Later on, I was able to defend myself and say to myself, "Wait a minute, is it really realistic to believe that I'm going to be thinking about her leg when our baby is making her entrance into the world? No, of course not. Give yourself a break. Take it easy on yourself, buddy." Everything turned out fine. The nurse wasn't upset with me, she just told me what to do since I was a novice at birthing. An ambiguous, unresolved, and uncertain feeling lasted for another hour about messing up with Lynn's leg and causing damage to the baby.

Then, the time came for me to cut the umbilical cord. It seemed so odd to cut this rubbery, spongy thing that was attached to our baby daughter. I worried that I was hurting her when the scissors sliced through the cord. My anxiety about being responsible for another's well-being was present. *Don't worry, buddy, the doctor is telling me to cut it, so it must be OK. He is handing me the scissors! I have no choice but to do it. I'm not hurting her. The doctor would not let me. But this is her skin, a part of her body. No, don't even go there. You know it is just OCD rearing its ugly face, trying to make you feel worried about hurting her.* I did not acquire more uncertainty as a result of cutting the cord. (At least not yet.)

Boy (I should say girl), what an ideal exposure experience for someone who obsessed about hurting others, particularly those who meant a lot to me. With scissors in hand, a potentially dangerous implement, I cut the umbilical cord and we had a beautiful little baby girl. I did it! And we were very happy as tears flowed down our cheeks. A couple of hours later, Lynn wondered whether the doctor had allowed the nutrient-rich cells from the umbilical cord to enter the baby's body. Instead of taking this query and calmly looking back at the chain of events and coming to some reasonable conclusion, I instantly felt my anxiety elevate and thought anxious "What if . . .?" thoughts. Lynn's curiosity functioned as a trigger to heighten my anxiety. I did not follow the birthing plan Lynn and I had so carefully prepared. Hence, our baby daughter was not as healthy as she could be. I was so tired and emotionally defenseless against this sudden revelation that I assumed the worst. I began to think that catastrophic consequences would ensue. I sensed it was my fault since Lynn was in no state to think about anything.

Beware of times when emotions completely drive thoughts, for as we know, the thoughts are colored, or maybe completely distorted, by the affect.

In fact, I was not emotionally defenseless; it was simply a difficult time to attempt to cope with the feelings when I had been awake all night. I went back in my mind and remembered that the doctor had been holding up the cord before and during the time I cut it, thereby permitting the beneficial nutrients to enter the baby's body. That meant that the cells must have gotten to their desired destination. Clearly, the doctor and nurses knew what they were doing and were up-to-date on all the latest in labor and delivery, including this little matter with the umbilical cord. I felt compelled to go find information about how long it took the cells to pass into a newborn. In other words, my OCD was not yet satisfied that the baby had been properly taken care of. Lynn and I did have some information we had compiled during the pregnancy. However, I didn't read anything. Why? It was a checking compulsion, serving no function other than to reduce my anxiety. I still felt some anxiety. This was therapeutic.

As a new father, I obsessed about hurting our little girl Elizabeth. She was so tiny and fragile that it seemed too easy to accidently drop her, squeeze her too hard, or not support her head enough. It came as a great relief to me to know that my wife also experienced the same fears. After we talked, I was absolutely certain that all new parents had similar anxieties and thoughts when it came to handling a newborn.

Generally, after the birth, I endured a greater level of nervousness than someone without OCD. In addition, there was also a feeling that I needed to do something to make reparations (do compulsions) for any perceived wrongdoing. I tended to do rituals by reassuring myself a lot, saying things like, "Elizabeth is fine. She's not as fragile as I believe she is. She's not hurt. My goodness, if that little pressure upon my shoulder hurt her, there would be babies stacked up sky high in the hospitals." All the while, my body tensed up and fear gripped my heart. When I spoke to my wife about her anxieties, I got the sense that she also thought about worst-case scenarios and worried about Elizabeth's head moving more than she would have liked. She appeared to be able to move on though, letting go of these anxieties. Her anxieties did not increase like mine did, nor did they typically initiate a chain of anxiety-provoking thoughts, feelings, and behaviors. She didn't think a lot about avoiding picking Elizabeth up as I did. I was proud that I did not let this fear win.

Life had changed since I began to think about the incident (when the baby gently touched my shoulder). Similar to any "distant" obsession, my fear was that life would never return to how it was before the incident. This reminded me of September 15, 1982 and I felt more certain that life had changed for the worst. Perhaps, I irreversibly hurt the little one. This had never actually happened and, on some level, I knew it never would. Anxiety was a short-lived phenomenon and an overreaction to a perceived danger. Clearly, I overreacted to slight, subtle bumps and rubbing movements when I held or moved the baby. My OCD just happened to get activated this one particular time rather than another time. Why? I didn't know. At times, all sufferers experience symptoms without knowing a clear precipitator.

My response to my second child's birth two years later in 2000 was different; it was a little less anxiety-provoking. I was more relaxed and less apprehensive in general, even though there were complications that made the delivery anxiety-producing. The intensity and duration of my anxieties were less the second time around. As a "seasoned veteran" of one birth, I was more comfortable and familiar with the birthing process. I felt more comfortable at the hospital, yet I knew that any birth was never taken for granted. I told myself that the sonograms showed that the baby had developed well and I had confidence in the hospital and the doctor. Our doctor seemed competent; we had been to several appointments with her and felt as calm as could be expected.

We arrived at the hospital at the appointed time, seven o'clock in the morning. Two hours later, Lynn was in the delivery room. The induction began. Everything was going fine and obsessions were nowhere to be found. There was nothing to obsess about because all was gradually and smoothly going forward. Lynn's medication was working and the nurses reported that there were no problems. I was next to her holding her hand, running my hand over her forehead, and imagining what the gender of the baby would be. Furthermore, I was curious what the baby would look like.

Suddenly, Lynn writhed in pain and screamed for help. The baby had to be coming. I glanced over at the nurse who appeared calmer than I felt. The nurse placed a respirator on her face and said that it should help her to breathe easier. The nurse was concerned about Lynn's asthma. But, in fact, the respirator made it more difficult for Lynn to breathe and feel comfortable. I started focusing on my breathing and had to take deep breaths to calm myself.

The nurse hurriedly called the doctor. She said that the baby was ready to be delivered. We were waiting for the doctor to arrive so that the birth could go forward. Lynn was rolling from side to side and grimacing in pain. She tightened her hand when the waves of pain came. I wanted to do something, but felt that there was nothing I could do to help. That was not exactly true. I remained with her, wiped her brow, held her hand, and encouraged her to hang in there until the doctor arrived. I assumed that the doctor was traditionally and legally bound to be present. The doctor took forever to get there; five minutes seemed like an eternity.

I was growing increasingly angrier by the second. My wife was in more pain than I had ever seen anyone experience, but the doctor was not there. *What can I do? There's nothing I can do besides what I'm already doing? Did I cause the pain? Was there something I could have done to prevent it, or were there warning signs that a husband should have observed? Wait, this is ridiculous!! I am not going to get into this stuff. This is OCD and I am not going to give into it. My wife needs me now. I have got to remain strong and be one hundred percent there for her.*

Finally, the doctor arrived and took charge of the situation. She became angry at the nurse because she did not understand the reason that the respirator was needed. Neither did Lynn. She was shaking her head, obviously attempting to remove it from her face. However, despite the doctor's order, the nurse insisted that the respirator remain on. *She must know what she is doing. She had stated that she had worked at the hospital as a nurse for twenty years. I have a lot of respect for nurses; my wife is one. But my wife is not able to put up with the discomfort. Should I say anything? Who am I to tell the nurse what to do? I am her husband. I must say something.*

My OCD often flared up when I felt helpless to do something or help somebody. Fortunately, when I really needed to make a decision and act, I was usually able to do so. I allowed the professionals to do what they earned their living doing, and I did not say a word. It was disconcerting that the professionals did not agree about using the respirator. However they worked it out. It was nothing that I could have done anything about anyways. Who made me an experienced person in the delivery room? Moreover, I remembered that my clients and their parents who interfered with the treatment process and did not have faith in it typically did not improve. Others who permitted me to do my job and did what I requested of them were much more likely to get better. I felt helpless, but I was able to think my way through the doubting maze that my OCD was leading me through. I was feeling the anxiety, anxiety that anyone would have experienced in this situation. I was fully in the present and not obsessing about anything that I could or should have done.

The moment I had been waiting for finally arrived. My son Christopher was delivered and I was extremely proud, happy, and spent. The nurse cleaned him off and handed him to me wrapped in a blanket. It was a good thing that I did not suffer contamination symptoms because, as all babies, he was wet, sticky, bloody, and covered with amniotic fluid when he arrived. I said a silent prayer as I did when my daughter was born, asking God to make my son healthy and free from OCD or any other anxiety or emotional disorder.

My parental instinct surfaced, and it wanted the best for my child. *Please, God, don't let my children have OCD. Please let the non-OCD genes manifest themselves in them; make the OCD a recessive and not a dominant gene.* Tears streamed down my face while I looked at and handled my new son as a sacred object. I was not going to let this birthing experience feel incomplete and unresolved like the umbilical cord worry that surfaced when Elizabeth was born. *I told you that everything would be alright. Did the doctor allow my wife to give birth without any drugs? Here I go again . . . Stop it!!*

Without any warning, the doctor requested morphine and said that she needed to assure herself that the entire placenta was extracted from the body. Due to the amount of bleeding, the doctor believed that she needed to examine my wife internally. She put on a latex glove and reached her hand to where the baby had been just seconds before. My wife screamed with horror at the new assault on her body. Again, I felt helpless and out-of-control. I couldn't do anything and had to remain at a distance from the bed. The nurse encouraged me to stay with my boy and talk to my wife from that distance. Realizing that my proximity would help my wife as much as a slap in the face, I talked to her from across the room. The doctor could not remove the remaining part of the placenta. She stated that my wife might have to get a hysterectomy. The doctor asked for more morphine. The nurse said that she had four cc's. of the painkiller in the syringe.

Upon hearing about a possible hysterectomy and the incorrect dosage of morphine, my wife yelled, "four milligrams, not four cc's." The nurse had made a mistake and the doctor chastised her for erring. Four cc's. of morphine could have killed my wife, and she knew it. Sometimes it was more stressful to possess more knowledge of a subject. My heart skipped a beat while the scene played out right before my eyes. So much had happened so rapidly that I was numbed to the happenings surrounding me. Everything seemed surreal. I just wanted what was right for my wife and wanted the professionals -- about whom I was having some serious doubts -- to do what needed to be done, but in a painless and harmless way.

The nurses rushed her to an operating room. During the trip there, my wife cried and cried. She repeatedly implored the doctor not to perform a hysterectomy. Throughout this ordeal, I did nothing. I <u>could not</u> do anything. I knew this as everything was transpiring. Since I could not do anything to assist my wife or the medical professionals, I determined that my OCD was causing some of my soaring anxiety and obsessionality. I was naturally anxious about everything that was happening, but there was no sense in obsessing about the sequence of events or thinking about what I could or should do to watch out for my wife's welfare. That's why we were at the hospital.

Thankfully, the ordeal ended on a happy note. Lynn did not have to have a hysterectomy and the bleeding had subsided some. She would have to stay in the hospital since she lost much blood, but it was just a matter of a day or two before she could return home. Most importantly, the baby was safe and healthy. Well, I couldn't know or influence whether or not he would have health problems and what they would be. I couldn't do anything about that, either. Time would tell. I was not going to permit OCD to prevent me from achieving a dream by having a family. There were many worse conditions for a person to have, and treatment for OCD would only improve in the future.

Don't let OCD take hold when there is nothing you can do about a given situation. Feel anxious, but tell yourself that the doubt and uncertainty is OCD. Identify OCD, remind yourself that it is only OCD, and that it is nothing to obsess about. Maybe being concerned is adaptive, but OCD is not. There are many things in life that are uncontrollable; the more we try to control the uncontrollable, the more suffering will follow.

Chapter 12

MEDICATIONS

This chapter is a journal entry from the late 1990's.

It is two months after my second child was born. The past two days have revived memories of seventeen years of taking some type of medication for OCD. Over the years, I have tried roughly fifteen different psychotropic medications. Yesterday, I was very sedated, and today, despite the alarm clock being set, I slept for twelve hours and missed a doctor's appointment. This behavior is very unlike me. Typically, I'm a very responsible person who makes it on time to engagements that I have scheduled in advance.

I am sick and tired of feeling like a guinea pig. Don't get me wrong. I believe that OCD results from physiological anomalies, neurobiochemical predispositions, and learned behavior in response to the environment. Frequently, medication is a necessary treatment modality. Nature and nurture play an important part in the life of each individual. For some, nature is a more prominent contributor to the symptoms, and for others the environment is. There is never a complete one hundred percent nature or nurture cause in any one individual. Humans are just too complex for that to be the case. I do believe that medication is an important part of treatment for OCD, especially when the sufferer is experiencing high levels of depression and/or anxiety. Medication can be very helpful. I have taken some kind of medication for more than two decades, and it has generally boosted my mood and decreased my anxiety. I am aware when my medication levels are low in my system. Anafranil (Chlorimipramine) has a short half-life and leaves the system quickly. If I do not take it on time, I feel terrible.

Recently, I have experienced very high levels of anxiety and my doctor has scrambled to come up with some medication that can help. Unfortunately, in the age of managed care, psychiatrists have become medicine managers, people who prescribe medication and have little time to establish any rapport with the patient. How much rapport is it possible to build during a fifteen minute office visit?

I have had four managed care physicians over the years and they are very similar. Basic knowledge about medications and past experience with psychiatrists has molded me into my own advocate. I have to ask them if I should administer the medication with or without food, take it in the morning or at night, how quickly it's supposed to work, and if it's OK to take with all the medications I'm already taking. In short, doctors may tell you very little about the medication that you are taking. Either the information I'm asking for (which seems important to me!) is deemed insignificant, or the fifteen minutes have run out. I think I know the answers to many of my inquiries, but it certainly would be more reassuring to know that the doctor is on top of things.

Today, I feel very tired and the medication forced me to take two naps. Everyone knows that kind of tired feeling, when their mind and body are exhausted to the point that it seems that nothing they do will revive them. I really hate this. I am aware that the medical community helps millions of people with pharmacotherapy. However, at times, I resent what seems to be many doctor's attitude of needing to justify their existence. If there is the least bit of symptomatology present, their training spurs them into action to immediately eradicate any "abnormalities." That's all well and good, but how about the clients? Encouraged to try different medications for the same problems, many of us begin to feel like walking pharmacies. Looking at all the pills that are prescribed for me right now, I am shaking my head. It gets to the point of absurdity. I am doing quite well on my current medication regimen, but my doctor, after hearing that I'm still obsessing a little, something that I've done for twenty years, wants me to try yet another medication to rid myself of all remaining obsessions. I do not know anything about this drug, but I'm still supposed to jump on the bandwagon. The medication is Serzone, a new weapon in the prescriber's chemical arsenal.

Before my current irritation surfaced about my medications, I went to see an OCD medication specialist, a psychopharmacologist who is current and familiar with all OCD medicines and any combinations of them that might be efficacious. I work with people with OCD and am very familiar with the medications that people take for the condition. This doctor and I collaborated and discussed my current situation in depth. This doctor suggested taking Anafranil with Prozac (Fluoxetine) and Klonopin (Chlorazepam) at a low dose if I felt that I wanted any more relief. This sounded reasonable. Anafranil is an OCD medication that's been around for a number of years. I've been on Anafranil before and it did help. This bit of success was good to keep in the back of my mind as a reference.

When the managed care physician suggested trying a new drug, as he had many times before, I said "yes" as I always had. I mentioned what the other doctor had recommended, but he had some reservations due to the possible side effects of Anafranil, such as drowsiness. He told me that I would be on such a low dose that it shouldn't affect me. In any case, I would gradually increase the dosages. I could always stop if adverse reactions emerged. He thought that a new drug, Serzone, had potential without the possible side effects. OK, I could buy this and I tried it. Much to my chagrin, and despite my hopes, it didn't work. In fact, it has knocked me for a loop for two days. Bad experiences such as this diminish one's confidence in medication.

It appears to me that as long as a brand new medication is available (and they always will be), my doctor wants me to try it. For him, the presence of one symptom requires immediate intervention. If something "may" help me, let's try it. I have not yet achieved a non-anxious nirvana state so let's keep popping those pills; one of them has to be right. Like others before me, I have finally reached the end of the line with experimenting with the medications. I have played that game long enough. Now they can find other people to try their new products on.

Recently, the press reported that there was some evidence that suggested that some of the SSRI medications (OCD selective serotonin reuptake inhibiting medications, e.g. Prozac, Luvox, Zoloft, etc.) might even generate suicidal thoughts in sufferers. (**As of 2007, there has been some research showing that this is not the case.**) I have heard the controversy since Prozac arrived on the market in the late 1980's and I have always believed that the people who did attempt to commit suicide and the ones who actually killed themselves were people who would have behaved similarly even if they were not taking the SSRI. The parents I talk to are understandably very concerned about their children taking SSRIs. As a parent, I would think twice myself. On the other hand, medications have helped millions of OCD sufferers. (There is now some data that show that these medications aren't dangerous to take.) I believe that medication, if needed to jump-start CBT, or required due to the severity of the OCD, remains a vital weapon fighting OCD. Because of the current frightening information that applies to a very, very small minority of clients who take SSRIs, keeping a very close eye on a young person's behavior is warranted now more than ever. Do not immediately discard the notion of medication because of the recent data that has surfaced. *I'm telling them to do something that can potentially bring them harm. How can I live with myself if anything horrific happens? I am telling them to make sure that they are in very close contact with the psychiatrist, and that they need to be aware of changes in their children's behavior and to report them to the psychiatrist. I . . . That's it! I'm getting outside of my head and going on with life. OCD tried to get me, but no . . . no . . . it is not going to. I won't let it. If OCD had its way, this book would never get published.*

Returning to my anger with the doctor, I couldn't fathom the nerve of my psychiatrist! He phoned and stated that he received my message concerning how sedated I was the previous weekend. This guy has the chutzpah to report that a lower dose is necessary to adjust the body to the presence of the medication. Now he tells me! I spend an entire weekend feeling as though I belong on the set of "Dead Man Walking," and he cavalierly relays the message that, "Oh, we goofed (He goofed!). We have to start slower."

This guy (I'm angry, so he has lost his professional title for the time being) must not realize what psychoactive medications can do to an individual (although he obviously should!). He's out playing golf and I'm shvitzing like an Airedale. The attitude of some doctors is what bothers me the most. The system that they helped develop and maintain isn't any better. I don't feel like a person, a human being, in this man's office, or for that matter, in any managed care psychiatrist's office. To them, I am an object upon whom to try their newest chemical acquisitions. I am not an object nor should I be subjected to this attitude and stance that certain HMO doctors seem to take. After the doctor suggested that I try the same medication at a lower dose, I felt very strongly that I had reached the end of my pharmacotherapy rope (and felt like I would have liked to hang the doctor with it).

After much reflection and a few months to calm down, I am now taking Klonopin, an anti-anxiety medication that helps to defuse the anxious powder kegs that go off in my brain from time to time. In combination with individual and group therapies, and with lots of personal reflection and support from my wonderful wife, the medication has allowed me to laugh at situations that had only caused pain and suffering before. I have gained a new perspective and now clearly see the unreasonableness and excessiveness of an obsession. Medication is not a cure, for I still have OCD symptoms; however, it allows me to function on an even keel more often.

I am a CBT therapist and treat individuals utilizing this orientation. However, I now know that when anxiety persistently and pervasively reaches an elevated level, it may be prudent to consider medication. I see both sides of the treatment continuum, knowing that the combination of biological and cognitive-behavioral modes of treatment often result in greater happiness and health. As a CBT therapist, clients frequently attribute their improvement to medication rather than CBT. It is frustrating to feel that my work, and the client's hard work, is not given the credit it's sometimes due. Because of the proliferation of medications for just about everything these days, I guess it's easier to give a pill credit than it is a change in behavior (though they both change brain chemistry). Like most, I want to do as much as I can without medication. I want to take credit for my diligent exposure work. Some people don't even require medication for an optimal outcome. Unlike some, I realize when my internal coping resources have been tapped to some depth and I require a psychopharmacological boost. There is nothing weak about this position. It is empowering to recognize one's limits. In reviewing these series of episodes and my treatment regimen, I am still taking Prozac and Klonopin. I would now be willing to try something new if my medication was not working well. I do not want the reader to think that the very difficult times I went through in this chapter mean that I would discourage trying appropriate medications.

In my view, it is important to find a doctor with whom you feel comfortable and who is knowledgeable about pharmacological treatments for OCD. After locating an experienced doctor, do not be afraid to try new medications. Despite my preceding diatribe, the stream of consciousness at that specific time in the past, I would always try something new if my medications were not working sufficiently. Most importantly, do not be afraid to be an informed consumer and an advocate regarding your own treatment.

Also, try to find a psychiatrist who has an appreciation for all empirical treatments, including CBT interventions. Despite evidence from numerous studies indicating that a combination of CBT and medication is the most effective treatment for OCD for most sufferers, a small number of uninformed, unenlightened doctors stand firm against CBT in favor of medications alone or combined with insight-oriented (analytic) treatment.

Chapter 13

OBSESSIONS AND COGNITIVE-BEHAVIORAL THERAPY (CBT)

Soon after hiring me, my employer asked me if I wanted to work with a couple of obsessive people. He believed that I had a good handle on the treatment of such individuals. Well, I should! I'm surprised that there isn't a picture of me in the dictionary next to the word "obsessive," and astounded and perturbed that I'm not the spokesperson for the cologne "Obsession." In this chapter, I am going to emphasize obsessions and internal experiences since I have a profoundly personal understanding of them. I will also discuss the treatment of such personal experiences.

The phenomenology of the obsessive individual with OCD continues to be difficult for the professional community to tap into. It's hidden, invisible, and unobservable. The only guide that the professional community has at its disposal is descriptions by obsessive people themselves.

To define what an obsession is, I will elaborate upon both others' and my internal experiences. An obsession generally differs from a neutral thought (i.e., "Today is September 19") in many ways. By definition, an OCD obsession is anxiety-provoking. Very infrequently, an obsession can be emotionally neutral. This means that the thought itself is not anxiety-provoking, though the long-term presence or personal reaction from having the thought may be anxiety-provoking. For example, someone thinks about numbers that flood his or her mind, or a song that invades and permeates his or her brain for several days or even months. The content of the obsessive thoughts are emotionally neutral, but frequently the presence of these bothersome thoughts cause anxiety. An obsession even differs from negative thoughts like, "I hate myself;" similar statements tend to be depressogenic and not anxiogenic. The obsessive thoughts, "I'm going to drop this baby," "Maybe there is some blood on this door handle," and "Let me check to see if the oven is still on" are common. OCD obsessions are much more frequent, longer-lasting, intrusive, distressing, and painful than other types of thoughts. Most importantly, they can lead to compulsive, ritualistic behavior, or an avoidance of the desired behavior.

Prevalent obsessions that often lead to compulsive behaviors and avoidance frequently originate from what I call the "Holy Trinity" of OCD: sex, violence, and blasphemy.   Because these subjects are sometimes scary, emotionally-charged, and unacceptable to think about, they prove to be fertile ground in which obsessions can grow.   For instance, what if a person had a lightning bolt thought that said, "I want to have sex with my sister." A sufferer might become anxious about the presence of the thought and do whatever he or she could (i.e., pray in a certain manner, think an opposite thought, etc.) to alleviate the anxiety.   This thought can take on greater meaning and be very frightening; no one, whether a sufferer or not, wants to have the aversive thought. An example of a violent obsession is, "I want to hurt that little girl." Again, a very provocative statement that almost begs for some sufferers to be obsessed about.   And religion can get very tedious for sufferers if they believe that they are sinning by having any sexual or violent thoughts.   Random thoughts are a part of the human experience; we all have meaningless, way-out-there, and bizarre thoughts on occasion.   OCD sufferers make more of them; they overanalyze their thoughts, too.   This is less difficult to do because the thoughts "stick" in an OCD sufferer's mind.

Here is an examination of another obsession. The thought, "I'd better lock the front door" functions as an adaptive response to the possibility (no matter how slim) of danger (crime or violence). People who live in cities and suburbs know that locking the door is taking a reasonable precaution. This particular thought likely leads to adaptive action (i.e., locking the doors one time) given the relative importance of the subject. But a person who obsesses, and doesn't only think casually about locking the front door, is literally repeating the thought in his head over and over again. Anxiety causes this repetition. He or she feels compelled by anxiety and obsessive thoughts to rethink the thought and to maladaptively double check to make sure the door is locked, even though he or she doesn't want to and would rather be doing something else (like sticking needles in his body!). With OCD, excessive anxiety functions as the motivator to act. On the contrary, when a neutral thought is not repeated many times, reason functions as the cause of action. Of course, every incident of checking the door is not a result of OCD or anxiety. From time to time, everyone goes to see whether a door is shut due to sheer curiosity and concern, not high levels of anxiety.

The obsession "The door may not be shut," or "It is not shut" may haunt a sufferer, hovering over him or her like dreary rain clouds. It seems that nothing that the person does can assist him or her to let go of this thought and its accompanying anxiety. He or she can keep busy doing activities, and this may work to distract the mind from the obsession. However, after completing the activity, he or she returns to the starting point, in the thick of the obsession.

It's not a matter of willpower or a lack of intelligence that causes a sufferer to act (ritualize) on his or her obsession. It's a matter of comfort and doing what is typically natural for humans to do, to act for short-term gain or reinforcement. Sufferers need to learn how to be more comfortable being uncomfortable. Only until they are able to do this will they reap the benefits of increased happiness and decreased anxiety for the long-term. Keep in mind that the goal of E/RP is not to eliminate anxiety, feelings of guilt, and other "negative" emotions. The goal is to experience a wider range of emotions, to experience all of life in its beauty, ugliness, and greatness, and to learn how to persevere, no matter what the circumstances are.

To that end, CBT asks the sufferer to experience some anxiety (experience the obsession) without engaging in compulsive acts or avoidant behavior that strengthen the ritual. This is E/RP. Feel the fear and don't do anything (ritual, avoidance) to reduce the strength of the fear. OCD is a trap that people fall into, an illusion that beckons, and a powerfully seductive force that can live and grow only with one's cooperation. CBT helps people to climb up and out of the snake-filled pit where a person might get bit.

Sadly, E/RP does not always help the sufferer. Common reasons why treatment for OCD does not work are: lack of motivation, secondary gain (reasons why people would not consciously and often unconsciously really want to improve, such as not having to work and feeling less stress due to lowered expectations of the family), lack of familial support, and stopping treatment before high-anxiety stimuli are confronted. Clearly, the entire onus is not placed upon the sufferer for improvement; the professional also must be competent and creative in providing proper treatment. Professionals in the mental health field make mistakes just like anyone else in any other line of work. Nevertheless, people entering treatment need to know that if one or more of the above factors has not been resolved before entering treatment, the professional will have a more difficult time helping the client. CBT practitioners are well trained in techniques of motivation and attempt to work with or recommend that the sufferer or his or her family get the necessary adjunctive assistance. Issues of secondary gain can be worked with and education is given to the client to let them know that early termination may mean unacceptable continued levels of anxiety.

Here, I will examine how CBT treatment helps me. The following journal example illustrates how obsessions can cause confusion and feared negative social outcomes. Other journal entries will also be examined later in the chapter to clarify what an obsession is and what appropriate treatment might look like. Since I was diagnosed at the age of fourteen, I have written sporadically in my journal.

My wife and I were at our neighbor's house at 1:00 P.M on a Saturday. They were kind to invite us over and prepare lunch for us. They were from Bolivia and spoke varying degrees of English. I spoke Spanish proficiently; we both took opportunities to learn about each other's language and culture. One neighbor said something and I smiled. I thought to myself, "Should I have smiled? Does he think that I am laughing at his pronunciation of an English word?" Immediately, I felt dry. My lips stuck together, which made it an effort to pry my mouth open. All moisture vanished from my body. My mind became very foggy and confused. Physiologically, this was my common reaction to uncertainty. My OCD light switch had turned on. I projected my anxiety onto them; I was already anxious about my command of Spanish, and it was easier to think that someone else had anxious feelings other than me. As a result, it was difficult to feel the anxiety. Perhaps my neighbor worried about what he said. Maybe I said something rude or crass without knowing. Projection was frequently my defense mechanism of choice.

In my "dry obsessional" state, it was much more onerous to think clearly and be and feel comfortable with the accuracy and correctness of each word. I turned into a human prune. As I experienced all the emotional and physiological changes, I started conversing with him again, though I did hesitate ever so slightly to process and adjust to my newfound murky internal state. It seemed that my mind was searching for verification of my anxiety. Every one of his facial movements, no matter how subtle, could be interpreted as an indication that he misinterpreted my behavior. Trying to make sense of what transpired, my mind scanned internally and externally for any clues, helpful or not, to resolve the entire issue. In retrospect, my mind had a very difficult time living with the uncertainty of whether or not my neighbor misattributed hurtful motives to my actions. My perception of the size of my smile was likely exaggerated. I doubted my perception of the incident, too.

One must remember that feelings are not facts. Just because I was anxious didn't confirm that they were offended. It didn't necessarily mean that they weren't, either. However, many of us sometimes take feelings at their face value and do not scrutinize what thoughts we have that may be contributing to the negative, painful feelings. Feelings, especially anxious feelings, are sometimes false alarms that take our attention away from what is actually going on. At my neighbor's house, I was aware that my elevated anxiety was due to OCD and not to the situation. My "Spanish OCD" had occurred before. I wondered what caused humans to become anxious for no sensible reason.

Rationally, I knew that my obsession about messing up socially and causing another person discomfort was unfounded. We had a good relationship with the neighbors and there was no real evidence during the conversation that I offended him. Despite my reasoning, the obsession lasted until the end of our conversation. It simply ran out of steam while I was looking and talking to my neighbor. Thankfully, anxiety does decrease over a relatively short period of time when an exposure is done and one remains in the situation.

The origins of anxious and fearful feelings harken back to a time in our evolutionary past when it was very useful to possess anxious feelings that led to quick, effective, goal-directed behavior that ensured our safety from predators. In short, when danger arose, the person either prepared to fight or fled the scene.

Of course, bad incidents still occur today, but they are not usually part of our daily existence. Although man has moved up the food chain, our nervous systems have not changed much (if at all) from our early forebears. The conditions under which a large segment of the world's population lives have changed dramatically. We do not have to go on a dangerous hunt for food; we are fortunate to have reasonably safe supermarkets and malls. Moreover, we are not generally stalked and sought after as prey by other animals. Humans are the hunters and we do not have to be perpetually vigilant. We do not have to be as anxious as we once had to be.

Individuals with OCD possess a central nervous system (CNS) that still activates when in the presence of non-threatening internal and external stimuli and cues. The switch is on when it should be off. Sufferers feel a compulsion to act even though every fiber of their being screams differently. CBT recalibrates the CNS so that one's excessive emotional reactivity lessens. On an "anxious day," sufferers might feel as compelled to ritualize as a mother does when her child is in immediate danger of being hit by a car. Other "less anxious days" may bring feelings equivalent to how a mother may feel if her child was walking while ten yards away from traffic. Clearly, when parents act to prevent a tragedy, it is an adaptive response to danger. On the other hand, when someone washes his or her hands for thirty minutes to remove any microscopic particle of gasoline after filling up the car, it does not represent an adaptive response.

One week after the "Spanish OCD" incident, a good example of overanalyzing the contents of my mind presented itself. It was another Saturday, a typical day in my life and in my OCD life. I didn't have to work so I had plenty of time to write a journal entry.

Today, when I woke up, I felt a little emotionally hung over from working many hours with tough, complicated clients for the past two days. After getting dressed, I went to run errands to the bank and the grocery store. While coming home from the grocery store, my mind automatically and persistently searched for something to grab hold of and keep. As usual, my mind felt uncomfortable roaming free without an obsessional "framework" and "anchor." I liked feeling that everything was fine, but my mind was not calm and satisfied.

Reading the newspaper while eating was a non-OCD morning ritual of mine. It reported that Ben Hogan died the day before, and half of the sports page was dedicated to his life. I focused on the first article at the top of the page. Golf was an interest of mine, and I wanted to understand and remember the contents of the piece. Sometimes my mind scanned for trivial information and tried to remember it. I missed the year in which he won three major championships. Then, I hesitated an imperceptible split-second, not knowing what to do. I wanted to practice what I preached and experience discomfort. I heard myself admonishing my clients to confront their anxiety and then live with forgetting, not knowing, letting go, and moving on. I kept reading the article; I did not go back to find the year. Next, I questioned whether I was truly anxious and wondered if going back was a ritual. Knowing this mental routine from the past and wanting to clear thoughts from my mind, the velocity of the psychic chatter accelerated. I analyzed whether I tried to take the "perfect" approach in handling this situation. Finally, in the face of much vexation and distress, I glanced back three lines and spotted the year. My anxiety went down. I became frustrated at myself because I looked back to ritualize. I had acted in a non-therapeutic way. The rest of the article didn't seem so valuable and worthwhile anymore. I concluded that OCD focused on the minor detail, signaling that if I didn't know that birthdate, I might as well stop reading. Continuing for no apparent reason, comprehension appeared to require more energy now. Mental absorption did not occur at the same rate as before I got into this crazy, absurd stuff with the article. I was obsessing about the contents of my mixed up mental state and doubting if I had acted in the most therapeutic way, even though rationally I knew I hadn't. I was angry because of my overthinking and not doing the "right" thing, continuing to read despite my anxiety.

I resumed reading and practiced forging ahead no matter what, realizing that by reading I was keeping my mind busy on things other than my mental rituals. Treatment had taught me that all-or-nothing thinking was not helpful; I could not believe that ritualizing only one time was akin to total failure. This was not true. I liked that I was attacking the OCD head-on. I felt better knowing that I was practicing E/RP. The number of obsessions and mental compulsions faded.

Whenever I begin to sink deeper into murkier OCD waters, I first recognize the fact that it is OCD. And OCD is an overreaction. In this case, it was a desire to be one hundred percent thorough; I had a fear of incompleteness that would lead to much discomfort. My analytical thoughts were actually covert (mental) rituals. I told myself that my mental energy was wasted on this unproductive stuff. The repetitive mental chatter served no good purpose other than to function as a compulsion. I had tried to reduce my anxiety by thinking a lot. But, I had to **feel** anxiety in order to reduce anxiety in a beneficial manner. CBT encourages sufferers to feel anxiety and discomfort rather than analyze anxious situations. When I feel a sense of incompleteness, I know that I am thinking and feeling in the most beneficial way.

I remember when my first and longstanding psychiatrist used to say that he always knew when I was going overboard with my obsessions. He said that sometimes I obsessed about obsessing. This was a clear indicator that my mind was consumed by unnecessary thoughts that appeared to feed off of each other, maintaining very uncomfortable thought patterns. (By the way, this is precisely why there is no evidence to support the use of psychoanalysis and psychoanalytic psychotherapies to specifically treat OCD symptoms. These therapies, though very useful at times, only serve to expand intricate internal worlds wherein obsessions, mental rituals, and OCD thinking are reinforced.)

Another journal entry took place a few weeks later at the start of winter. I dressed so that I could go outside and get the newspaper. The distance that I had to travel to retrieve the newspaper was directly proportional to the "bad weather index." I was beginning to believe that the delivery person carried measuring tape to preserve this equation, confirming that the newspaper was indeed further away from the house when weather conditions worsened. Anyway, as I approached the door to go outside, I asked myself the natural question, "Was I presentable to the outside world?" I sometimes had this sixth sense that people were watching me when I was outside. I was not paranoid, people really were. No, no, that was not true. It just seemed that way when I was highly anxious. My first psychiatrist called this tendency to worry about what people could be thinking about me in public "self-referential thinking." For me, it was a sub-clinical form of social anxiety.

The difference between other people and me was that I had to answer my own question about being presentable. I had to really answer it so that I knew I had answered it so that I felt comfortable getting the newspaper. I had to think thoughts like, "I look fine, good enough for going outside. Yes, all my clothes are on. So what if my hair is sticking up a little. Sure, the clothes don't match, but who cares?" I had to think and feel a certain way while entertaining these thoughts. Sometimes repeating the sentences in my mind aided in reducing my anxiety. The consequence of not asking and not responding to these questions was that, while venturing outside to gather the newspaper, I would have felt very anxious and uncertain about my appearance, even though I knew on some level that I was suitably attired. The fear (or obsession) was appearing inappropriately dressed (or undressed!), thus not acting sexually appropriate. This would mean others might encounter my perceived perversity and lack of control and awareness about a basic behavior like dressing. The compulsion was to reassure myself in a certain way. E/RP therapy requested that I go outside in various states of anxiety-inducing incomplete and sloppy dress to elevate my anxiety without using the usual self-reassurance. I needed to feel "not quite right" when leaving to go outside. I practiced thinking that my hair was messed up when I left the house. I desensitized to this experience after multiple trials.

After waking up groggy in the morning, anyone may feel the same way about walking outside. However, the anxiety that I am talking about varies from most people's anxiety. It is more intense and consuming. The thoughts and feelings take on a life of their own, bothering me like an extremely stubborn, persistent, and annoying person. It is as if a light switch turns on in my head. I feel very strongly compelled to turn it off by continuing to answer my queries. Engaging in mental rituals also assists me in calming down and reducing my internal level of stimulation. The world will be fine and I can go on enjoying the day. The only thing that I have to do is to tell myself that my hair is fine. That's it! What's the big deal?

The big deal is that, once a pattern is established that requires a person to think or feel a certain way before acting, the person becomes a slave to his or her thoughts and feelings. Sometimes we're not going to feel like thinking the "prescribed" thought (mental compulsion) before going outside. Other times we are not going to think it in the "right" way. Yet other times, we might not feel "good" about how much we emotionally experienced the entire episode. As all experienced sufferers know, ritualizing makes us feel comfortable for the short-term. During the process of trying to organize thoughts and feelings in the mind, individuals may begin to obsess about performing rituals. At this juncture, anxiety has spiraled around, thoughts become unclear, and feelings are numbed or blunted. Follow the same procedures outlined previously in this chapter to escape the OCD trap when overthinking and mental compulsions try to take control.

During the next summer of 2001, I attended a practice round at the United States Open golf tournament. This journal article is from that day. For a guy who felt overresponsible for everything, I could only look back and smile at some of the moments of anxiety that I experienced there. The most memorable and noteworthy occurred when I was watching the young phenom Tiger Woods play the ninth hole. He hit a monster drive on a very long six hundred yard par five hole. The crowd egged him on to attempt to hit the green with his second shot. All of the other golfers were leaving their second shots fifty to one hundred yards from the green. There were two reasons for this: they could not hit it that far; and/or they did not want to risk landing in a very deep valley in front of the green. Tiger obliged the crowd by pulling out a fairway wood and trying to reach the green. His ball went a little to the right, but it had the distance. There were some people in the area where the ball was going. Not until the ball was almost there did someone yell "Fore!," the universal golf "heads up" signal.

As Tiger was walking down the fairway to his ball, I had a strange sensation that something was not quite right. Just as someone yelled to warn others about the incoming projectile, I felt uneasy and unbalanced as if something was askew. It wasn't anything psychotic. I wasn't having delusions or hallucinations, and I knew what was happening to me and around me. I felt that something had to be erased or corrected. I started fearing that my inaction had led to something bad happening to another. I wondered if I had heard someone yelling because he or she got hurt when the golf ball hit him or her. Spectators in the crowd nearby probably talked loudly and it had nothing to do with anyone yelling or getting hurt. Very high anxiety caused my perceptions to verify my feelings, even though I thought that what I had heard was not a shriek of pain. Next, I began to question whether I had "properly and adequately" thought about, and experienced, the whole scene. My imagination functioned on overdrive, inquiring internally about the possibility that maybe this was not an OCD phenomenon. I thought that maybe I really should have felt badly about not warning others. Maybe, feeling bad was an adaptive response; perhaps, it was partially my fault that the warning came late and someone may have gotten hurt. It was terrible to feel as though I could have prevented something from occurring and feeling angry and frustrated because I didn't do enough. I was dumbfounded why I didn't yell (in spite of the presence of hundreds of others watching the scene). It must have been all my fault.

I was aware what this was all about. It wasn't anything new. It was the same tired old theme that had been harassing me for at least a decade, the overresponsibility theme. This unsettled and apprehensive feeling continued to float around and colored everything that happened to me for the next thirty seconds.

Whenever this happens, I can do a few things. I can acknowledge that this is an OCD feeling and resume what I am doing, exposing myself to anxiety. Or I can keep acting without consciously admitting that this is OCD. I have concluded that either path I choose to take results in therapeutic action since exposure occurs in both scenarios.   There were no OCD anxiety-reducing behaviors there.   It was a win-win situation; both choices led to helpful outcomes as long as I didn't ritualize (i.e., try to convince myself emotionally that I was not responsible for the golf ball going where it did, or asking someone if another person had been hurt).   An OCD sufferer can not emotionally convince him or herself of anything even if they rationally know the reality of the circumstances.

The next journal entry came from a psychotherapy session a week after the U.S. Open Golf Tournament. Here, I will look at treatment in the context of helping someone else with E/RP

A man revealed that he was preoccupied and petrified about "bad" things happening to him. A "bad" thing ranged from forgetting his wallet to someone in his family dying. He had not experienced enough of life to realize that most "bad," unpleasant, inconvenient incidents make us uncomfortable; nevertheless, we get through them, obtain the necessary help, and move on with our lives. Just the idea of something "bad" happening to him raised his anxiety significantly. Why was he fearful of "bad" things happening? He talked about being a very sloppy, careless youngster who, later in life, made a decision that he did not want to live his life that way. He could not recall anything else that had influenced or transformed him from being a careless person to a slow, compulsively careful person.

It was clear to me that his perception of his past was skewed by his present experiences. Any current example of compulsivity must have reminded him of his past disorganization as a youngster. However, I believed that the difference was minute compared to his analysis that there was a huge chasm between what his behavior had been and how it manifested now. Anxiety and perfectionism can distort not only your sense of the present, but of the past as well. Everybody's memories are notoriously poor; anxiety adds another layer of cloudiness to them.

A couple of weeks prior to this session, I told him that if his car broke down, it would serve as a great opportunity for him to practice problem-solving skills and to tolerate the anxiety that he felt since something did not go as planned. How many times had things not gone as planned in my life? Yes, that was correct, on a daily basis. To be fully alive and functioning at one's optimum level, one had to take small, calculated risks. Driving on the interstate was dangerous. On the flip side, it was also the fastest, most convenient way to get from one location to another. In the vast majority of outings nothing terrible occurred. There were no guarantees for a smooth, uneventful trip. I encouraged him to drive and behave with reasonable precautions (i.e., driving defensively and at the speed limit).

I provided this man a choice. He could choose to live with all the inherent risks that life entailed, or he could be paralyzed with anxiety and indecision and be dependent upon his parents for basic necessities for a long time. I did not pull any punches with him.

This man's complex clinical picture included more than OCD. It didn't make sense to him to even commit very little, innocuous errors to get used to the discomfort he experienced. There was more present that was not anxiety-based and interfered with him engaging in E/RP. I asked him to pretend that he did not bring a wallet to a store, and instead, ask me for money at the counter to purchase an item. He did not understand the rationale behind this therapeutic exposure technique. If he was going to live his life trying to prepare himself to never forget anything, to always appear the same way, to never be late, and to make no mistakes, no wonder he had so many problems.

Moreover, he also talked about being scared of what he called a deja vu feeling that he experienced sporadically. For instance, while watching television, if he foresaw a Dial soap commercial coming on and it did appear on the screen, he would experience much anxiety. He didn't really believe that the coincidence meant anything mysterious and sinister. Nevertheless, he couldn't shake a pervasive uncertain feeling whether he had some "supernatural" powers and could see into the future. Not that he would be responsible for someone else's death if he thought of their demise, but this would be the scariest thing for him to be able to foresee. He didn't want there to be **any** (not one in a million) chance of a connection between what he thought and what happened. In reality, of course, he could think whatever he desired and it would have no impact on the world. He misinterpreted and overreacted to coincidences. By acting like he did, he became more hypervigilant about the deja vu experiences, thus envisioning more when there weren't any additional ones.

Treatment consisted of continuously exposing him to situations in which he felt uncomfortable, starting with the less difficult events and moving on to the more difficult ones. As an aside, I never use the words easy or easier to describe an exposure. I say the words less difficult or least difficult. Facing fear is never easy. He needed to work his way up an anxiety hierarchy that the two of us created. By rating his anxieties to numerous stimuli and situations, we gradually climbed up the ladder when I exposed him to anxiety-provoking stimuli and situations. Concerning the deja vu experiences, I asked him to think about different products when he watched television, and if that product did by chance appear on the screen, to not erase or neutralize any uncertainty about the connection between his thought and what he saw on television. He needed to experience the anxiety, not avoid, escape, erase, or neutralize it. Doing the exposures provided him a beneficial direction to take. He could get better than he was. It was up to him.

It is always important to refrain from doing something to reduce anxiety. The more one wonders whether or not you should engage in anxiety-diminishing behavior, the greater the chance is that one will behave in that way. More time is available to talk oneself out of therapeutic action. Keep anxiety up and do whatever is necessary to not perform rituals. I have seen many people decide to do rituals after debating about it for one to two minutes. Anxiety reinforces anxiety; just do it (or Nike it) maintaining higher anxiety.

In this case, I believed that I didn't do enough refraining from ritualizing and didn't perform up to standards as a therapist. Maybe I didn't do enough helpful exposures. Perhaps I was not exposing him to his fear of death enough and not doing my best. Maybe I didn't know what enough was. Perhaps enough was not a useful abstraction. What was enough or my best? I didn't really know. I couldn't clearly and precisely define it. But it was evident that the vast majority of times when I was presented with a task to complete, I did work enough. I simply didn't feel that way at times. So what I did to help myself was to intentionally "make mistakes" in therapy. I wasn't disrupting treatment of others; I simply felt bad even though I had done enough (and usually more than that). I needed to expose myself to anxiety and all the other negative emotions that were experienced when I felt or thought that I had erred. For response prevention, I did not correct "my error" or reassure myself that the "mistake" was not that important.

Furthermore, when I was not sure whether I had done my best, I told myself that I may have not done well enough. The presence of doubt (with the word may) demonstrated that I was taking therapeutic action since may increased my anxiety more than any other word or words. I was aware that my perception of what a mistake "really" was was skewed; I realized deep down that I most likely did not "really" commit an error. Sometimes I tell myself that the reason that I have anxieties about goofing up is that I do care greatly about what I am doing. However, I don't need to feel high anxiety to be compassionate. My standards are higher, but I am not going to engage in OCD thinking. Caring to the point of obsessing is "too much of a good thing."

This discussion reminds me of a common statement that a sufferer makes during treatment. The sufferer says something equivalent to, "Something terrible will happen if I don't (or do) do that, I just couldn't live with myself if I hurt someone else by not doing enough." How many times have I heard this pronouncement and similar versions of it? The client's rationale for engaging in a particular behavior or sequence of behaviors is to guard against catastrophe. The individual feels that a dangerous, perilous outcome rather than a mere troubling, annoying one will ensue. It's no wonder that a person with OCD may avoid performing behaviors that increase his or her anxiety level and opt for the anxiety-reducing alternatives.

In response to the aforementioned statement of anxiety and dread, I tell my clients and myself, "Life is a messy, unclean, contaminated, unpredictable process that we either accept as such on some level, or we get stuck while doing things that temporarily help us feel more comfortable and in control of our fears." Then I tell my clients and myself, "Jump into the muck, murkiness, and uncertainty of life. This is the path towards living a full and happy life, and it provides us the best opportunity to do what we wish and follow our dreams.

Chapter 14

MY WORK

I have worked professionally with OCD sufferers for over ten years; a large percentage of my clients in my full-time practice have had a diagnosis of OCD. Over the years, I have met hundreds of sufferers. When I facilitated a support group for five years, I came to know some personally. Some individuals were more memorable to me because their OCD symptoms were more bizarre and unusual, though every person had a slightly nuanced clinical presentation. Everyone's OCD is different, and every family is different, as well. Many sufferers enlist the help of their family members to succor them by performing rituals or assisting them to perform their own rituals; families can unwittingly reinforce the OCD. This chapter will shed further insight into my experience treating others and their families, and the knowledge and wisdom I have gained will be explored.

Here is important background information that will help you to understand my perspective when confronted with a sufferer and his or her family. In graduate school, I learned the importance of knowing who I was and where I came from in order to optimally help others. Luckily, I grew up in a loving, stable, and consistent family environment. Notwithstanding that, it wasn't perfect, but I could have ended up with a much worse family in the adoption process. Before my graduate school experience, I thought this was the way most people lived. Boy, was I in for a surprise. The variety of individual and family experiences was enormous.

The best thing that my parents did was to disallow me to use OCD to circumvent normal, everyday routines and activities. Sometimes on the weekends during high school, I lay down on my bed to escape any unpleasant feelings I had. I remember my mother and father saying, "I know you feel awful, but you need to keep busy. Sometimes you just have to do things that you don't want or feel like doing." They were persistent in their efforts to get me moving. Fortunately, they were successful. I was not clinically depressed for much of this time, so getting out of bed was more of a possibility. I received the important message from them that **they believed in me,** and this extra vote of confidence in my ability to confront life and its challenges helps me to this day. In addition to believing in me, my family did not perform any OCD rituals or help me ritualize in any way. Since I didn't ask for reassurance, no one had an opportunity to reinforce my OCD. (I was good at strengthening it all by myself.) The faith that my parents had in me continues to be a wonderful blessing.

Unfortunately, some sufferers do not receive such a positive message from their families, and this is completely understandable. For many families, especially those who have assisted in reducing the anxiety-related OCD's grip, the pattern of comforting and nurturing at all costs is very difficult, but still very possible, to break. You ask, "What's wrong with comforting and looking out for the person?" Absolutely nothing, except when the support doesn't allow the sufferer to confront fears that they need to in order to improve. Families need to permit the sufferer to experience anxiety and discomfort when facing OCD, for if they do in the long run, they will enhance the person's confidence and ability to fight OCD. Families usually act in a caring manner. Families believe that their role is to behave according to comforting and caring principles. In the case of OCD, acting in the best interests of the sufferer is actually achieved by assisting them to actively attack the symptoms, or at least to avert helping in the avoidance or escape from fear. Ultimately, with the possible exception of younger children, the responsibility lies with the sufferer to change his or her behavior. The sufferer needs to do as much as possible to combat OCD. The family sometimes, with help from a therapist, can provide a home environment that is more conducive to desirable behavioral change. Paradoxically, generating or allowing anxiety to be present is a loving gesture that will truly help a person recover from OCD.

I have traveled to scores of sufferers' homes and have been privileged to meet them in their own environment. Homes are filled with cues (objects, memories, images, people) that often increase one's anxiety. No one wants his or her home to become "contaminated," unsettling, and unlivable. For most, your home is your castle (whether an apartment, condo, townhouse, single family house, or an actual castle). It is your refuge and sanctuary from the unpredictable, cruel, wonderful, terrible, forgiving world that we live in. However, a sufferer's home is almost always his or her worst OCD place. Everyone is at home more than any other place; therefore, there are more opportunities to become conditioned to feel anxious there.

It is not difficult to see why family members give into OCD. There are some challenging questions for which a sufferer might want an answer. For example, someone who is anxious about being "clean enough" might ask if they are sufficiently clean. They might ask OCD-related questions such as: "Did I take enough time in the shower?," "Did I use enough soap?," "Did you wash your hands?," "Do I smell?," "Do you see any dirt on my hands?," "Will you help me in the shower?," and, "Will you wipe me after I go to the bathroom?" As you can see, anxiety is a very powerful adversary. It can, if family members permit, make the sufferer dependent on others for basic hygiene tasks. When individuals do not feel self-sufficient anymore, an unhealthy pattern appears.

Even with the most innocuous questions about cleanliness, a helpful answer is (as long as it doesn't reduce anxiety), "You already know the answer to that question. It helps you when I don't answer." Sufferers need to know how best to act to weaken the OCD; this is done by resisting or at least postponing asking OCD reassurance questions to begin with.

Sufferers may make excessive and unreasonable behavioral demands on others to assuage their own anxiety. If followed, OCD rules govern the household. Typical examples of this include: "making" others wash their hands, "making" others get food for them, "making" others prepare different food only for them, "making" others keep "contaminated" objects away from them, or "making" others keep their distance (a person can be a contaminate) and never touch them or their belongings. Remember, OCD sufferers are typically sensitive, self-conscious, helpful people. OCD is "making" them behave differently than usual. I use "make" because it is the family's choice if they give into and follow the OCD rules that the highly anxious person feels compelled to observe.

I implore family members and friends to seek CBT if they are unable to refrain from performing reassuring, reconfirming behaviors. For maximum benefit (or sometimes almost any benefit), family and friends need to be on board. Most likely, sufferers know that what they are doing or asking you to do is reinforcing the disorder. The good news is that even if reassuring behavior has been maintained for many years, it can still be changed, and the sufferer, the family, and friends can lead happier lives. The majority of families who need assistance realizes that any disorder involves the entire family system that the sufferer lives in, and they agree to seek professional support. The family will function more smoothly with less tension and conflict if the family makes this wise decision. Sufferers may not thank you now, but they will for years to come. In fact, sufferers might become annoyed, irritated, and even angry because they are left to experience anxiety.

Anxiety is very uncomfortable, but it does not harm anyone. Asking reassuring questions may worsen before it improves; change is difficult for anyone. This is called an "extinction burst." When you try to modify behavior in a healthy way (by not answering reassuring questions at all and raising anxiety), it is natural that the sufferer will fight more fiercely for you not to change what you were already doing. But the situation will improve if you don't give in and answer these questions. Sufferers, request that your family members receive assistance if needed. It is in your long-term interest.

Healthier families allow others to learn about their patterns of interaction and are not averse to outside influences recommending changes; the sufferer and the family benefit from an exchange of information. Discussed here are two examples of families who did not act on this recommendation. They will help clarify and bring to light what happens in real-life situations, and why it is important to seek assistance. They will also demonstrate my reactions (including my OCD) to the two complicated cases and will provide suggestions regarding the most beneficial ways for the sufferer and the family to manage the OCD.

The first client had not improved to the extent that his parents deemed appropriate or reasonable, given the money and time involved. This bothered me, and I got a slight, dull headache whenever I thought of the parent's unhappiness. My response reflected my concern and attention to the case. I didn't want to obsess and beat myself up for any real or perceived errors on my part, yet the fear frequently asserted itself, making it very difficult to feel good about myself and what I had done with the case. All I wanted to do, and all I was going to do, was to observe what happened and not obsess.

The first case I'll describe concerns Jim, age twenty-three. During the initial consultation with my boss, while the parents described the young adult's problematic behavior, his mother burst out laughing about her husband's angry reaction to his son's description of his obsessions. He had intrusive, distressing thoughts of his father engaging in sexual intercourse with another woman. As a result, Jim needed his mother to perform a compulsion; she needed to say that the father was faithful to reduce his anxiety. (In this family, there was no adultery really occurring, only fear.) The symptom likely reflected the turmoil within the family. Obviously, the dynamic observed between the parents at the initial consultation signaled trouble. The client and his mother enjoyed laughing at the father's expense despite the sensitivity of the subject matter and the sad, helpless reaction that the father exhibited. My boss referred him to me and said that it was evident that the parents needed some help to assist their son. After learning about the case, my lips dried like they did when I became very apprehensive and anxious. I had an unsettled, unresolved feeling about the chances for treatment success.

A week after I got the case, I learned that the parents were contemplating separation, and this confirmed my belief that I was dealing with a disturbed family. In Jim's case, his mother encouraged the verbalization of an obsession (which occurred frequently in the household, the client would tell his father in front of his mother when he had an obsession about infidelity), and it only served to strengthen the undesired behavior because the mother promoted compulsive behavior. She told my client to reassure himself by asking his father if he had had an affair. Nothing exists in a vacuum -- not even OCD -- and the people that one lives with possess the greatest opportunity to effect change. My time with any client is short compared to the client's time with his or her family. Even my maximum of six hours per week of intensive work pales in comparison to the other one hundred and sixty-two hours that remain in the week.

From the beginning of treatment, I recommended that the parents receive supportive therapy from someone who could help them provide an environment more conducive to therapeutic change. This help was very important for this OCD sufferer and many others to gain the most from treatment. Depending upon the degree of reinforcement, treatment may be all but impossible without the family's help. The parents declined my recommendation and I went on treating him and doing the best I could. I agonized over this decision because there was no clear-cut answer to the question, "Is it better to stop, change the focus of treatment, or continue as before when the family was not fully cooperative and not taking a professional recommendation seriously?" My clinical judgment at that time was that the client was making enough progress to warrant continued treatment. I believed very strongly in CBT and wanted a fellow sufferer to receive the help he needed. As long as he was not completely sabotaging and undermining my work, I felt that I could still help him. Jim needed E/RP treatment, and I practiced interventions with him daily. I was very competent to help him.

I was reminded how difficult a family it was when the father called my boss, just two weeks after therapy began, and inquired why he hadn't yet observed any changes in his son. My hands started to shake slightly when my boss, despite being very supportive, relayed the family's message to me. The parent's expectations were very unrealistic, despite being bright, intelligent, and high-functioning professional people. OCD took time to grow; likewise, therapy took time to work.

However, my client persisted in demonstrating an unreadiness for and a resistance to treatment. He was willing to perform lower-level exposures, ones that did not make him very anxious. However, when asked to do medium-level exposures, he put his foot down and said, "No more." This course of action slowed down the progression of therapy considerably. I have learned that when people begin to dictate the pace of their own therapy, it is typically an ominous sign. The sign was accurate; he did not get much further in treatment.

I persevered, again requesting that his parents get help. It was a very delicate matter, asking and recommending that any parent receives help. These parents may have felt that I was blaming them for their son's problems. I had never said anything resembling this, nor would I ever because it wasn't true. Parents' defenses rise when there is talk about getting them help. They say, "The OCD is his problem. He is the one that has to change. Do something to make his or her symptoms better," (as though their child is a car and I'm a mechanic trying to fix him or her). The mother felt threatened and wondered aloud about how good a job she had done over the years with my client. She was certain that she had provided sufficient positive reinforcement, praise, and love for her son. I was not questioning that. I was simply saying that he needed his parent's help now with his OCD. He was not able to fully participate in treatment by himself, for two reasons. First, he was not ready for treatment and sufficiently motivated to get help. Second, his parents involved themselves in a significant number of OCD incidents. Everyone needed to be on the same page for the sufferer and the family to improve.

I have spoken about the objective facts of the case. Now, let's jump into the part that was murky and mysterious. My primary obsessional theme was the fear that I was not doing enough, and that perhaps I would be responsible for Jim not improving. You could see why this case was tailor made for me to obsess about. When working with clients, real human beings with real troubles, I did not want to cause any harm. In fact, I wanted to help. With my "overresponsible" OCD, it was easy for me to feel as though I was doing harm despite evidence to the contrary. I thought that I could have goofed at many steps in therapy. When anxious, there seemed to be too many ways of making a mistake.

I started thinking, and sometimes believing, that I should have done something differently. Since my interventions were not working, I jumped to the conclusion that it was my fault. Well, no it was not. *But is there something that I could have done differently, something that I missed in this case? What other therapeutic approach or technique might have worked?* The first thing that came to mind was when I was in a meeting speaking about the case to a colleague, and she mentioned that using yellow food coloring could act as a useful exposure stimulus for someone with a fear of being "contaminated" by urine. Jim had this fear. Mix the food coloring in water, touch it, and wipe it on clothes and skin. I had asked my client to do some other "contamination" exposures, and my colleague's idea caught me off-guard. Sure, I had heard about this technique before, and probably had even used it before. *So why had I not thought about it for this case? Is it too late to use this with my client? Does it really matter in the big picture? I'm having him do exposures, even though they don't involve food coloring. Is this the one exposure that would have made all the difference?*

I tended to immerse myself in the subtle nuances and minutiae of a case when I was in my obsessing mode. Even if there were important issues to think and talk about, it was easy to get caught up and have a harder time focusing on these overarching concerns, though fortunately I could when I needed to. For instance, it was important how I treated someone; the different techniques and strategies I employed were significant, and also were the crucial rapport and trust that developed. These were all pervasive, global issues in the case. However, focusing on details became unproductive when I beat myself up over not having presented an exposure on Tuesday and then doing it on Friday. The notion that I did not act soon enough, which I feared inevitably led to unintended catastrophic consequences, was blown totally out of proportion to the real effects of a trivial, almost nonexistent delay. It was ridiculous.

I also obsessed about not implementing a comprehensive incentive plan for this young adult. There was a very simple system implemented that allowed him to buy a comic book if he had performed a certain percentage of homework. Demand was high and his supply was low; it was a great time for this reward. Typically, I didn't immediately construct an elaborate reinforcement system with an adult, but sometimes I did, particularly if motivation was low and rewards for completing home assignments may have been helpful. This man kept telling me over and over about how motivated he was and about his diligent efforts practicing E/RP outside of sessions at home. I had no reason to disbelieve him. However, in retrospect, an incentive plan might have helped him make more progress. After this case, I became more careful about utilizing reinforcements with adults. I didn't think I did anything wrong, but being more cognizant of different factors that played a part in making that judgment helped. I saw and understood why I had acted the way I had.

Ultimately, Jim did resolve many of his OCD issues. However, family problems interfered with his ability to make a full recovery. The case reminded me that I could not force improvement upon the family. In spite of wanting more control of the case, the family was going to do what the family was going to do. I didn't believe that my OCD had any unhelpful effects on the case. I felt more anxiety working with this individual; however, my discomfort had no effect on the overall course and outcome of treatment. My anxiety did not manifest and express itself overtly. But, it did once when I regressed and urinated in my bed, a certain atypical and conspicuous (and smelly) sign of high stress.

People have always told me that I don't appear stressed, even when my subjective anxiety is very high. This assists me in treating anxious people. I do believe that during some cases I am more preoccupied with obsessive, compulsive, and self-doubting thoughts, but these thoughts have not interfered with treatment. When preoccupied, the worst that happens is that I don't react quite as rapidly (a matter of a half-second or so) to something someone says or does. My propensity is to speak and move a little slower than others anyway; that is my inherent, innate style. No one suspects or knows that OCD infiltrates my mind from time to time. I have improved in letting myself experience anxiety, talk about it, and act in therapeutic ways. My recommendation, no matter how repetitive and compulsive, is to practice always feeling the anxiety.

The second family OCD case that I will elaborate upon to increase awareness of the importance of familial support, and to provide strategies for sufferers and family members, was also an interesting, memorable one. I had met with Tom, a sixteen year-old teenager three times, and he had made it clear from the beginning that his father was not to be included in any way in his treatment. I was not to speak to him at all; the reason was vague to me. There was much animosity between the two and it appeared to Tom that avoiding his father was the best way to handle things. Like the first case, when a client tried to dictate treatment parameters, it was a dubious sign.

The fourth session began with Tom expressing much anger toward his father. He and his father had gotten into an argument within the past couple of days, and this venom came from that incident. Well, this wasn't your typical surly, angry adolescent. I knew one when I saw one. He alleged that his father was hitting him with an open hand. He had no marks on his arm, or the rest of his body, to prove his accusations, but he went on and on about various acts of mistreatment that he had suffered at the hands of his father. I told him that it was right for him to disclose private information to an adult he trusted. I told him that I had to keep confidentiality unless someone was in danger. Knowing that this client had a flair for the dramatic, I processed what he was reporting with some caution.

Saying that, when anyone makes these types of allegations, I am bound by law to take him or her seriously. I became extremely anxious about the prospect of having to report misbehaving parents. I could be responsible for the break-up of the family. *Wait a minute, just make the call and don't avoid the conversation.* I wasn't going to allow my "overresponsibility" theme take control and not to make the call. I called the county child protective services department about the case, but they said that it was not a reportable case since there was no concrete, visible evidence that pointed to the father. It didn't help the boy's case when he said that his father wouldn't even know his name if he walked into the room. This immediately raised doubts about the truth and accuracy of the information. Later in the session, he raised more flags when he wanted his mother to come into the room and hear what he had to say regarding his father's misbehavior. He stated that she didn't know anything about the incidents. At this point, the tone of his voice indicated that he was very upset. I sensed by his facial expressions, eye movements, and gestures that he had ulterior motives for inviting his mother into the office, and that there was something else he wanted. This turned out to be a correct assumption.

Needless to say, the session ended on a note that questioned whether OCD therapy should and would continue then, especially given what had surfaced in the session. Obviously, his safety was of paramount concern and needed to be the top priority. Tom's mother thought that her son was lying and that her husband had never hit him. His father had taken away his tennis privileges for one month for not completing his homework one night. His mother believed that he was using me to get what he wanted, more tennis time. The father's frustration and high expectations of his son, in spite of his son earning good marks in all his classes, caused him to excessively punish his son. The tennis court was a place that Tom visited every day; it functioned as a sanctuary away from the uncertainty and anxiety of the rest of his world.

I believe that the punishment should always fit the crime. Not to permit him to go to the tennis court for one day is still a form of punishment, but a reasonable one. The boy knew that a one-month punishment was meant to take away something that he valued tremendously, not only to teach him a lesson. The parents were right in knowing that taking away the privilege of playing would garner his attention since tennis was so meaningful to him. Where they misfired was in the number of days to take away tennis; the punishment did not fit the crime. I talked to the parents about this, explaining that a one month punishment would only lead to more anger and much less of a chance of any lasting behavioral change on the son's part. They would not yield. Before treatment could continue, I said that the parents needed to be more involved in the case. There were some problematic dynamics present within the family that had to be addressed so that treatment had a chance at a positive outcome. At that point, they took a break from treatment.

A few months later, after the family returned from their summer vacation, I received a phone call from the boy's mother. She wanted to set up an appointment for her son. Her son was starting school soon and she wanted to get him treated before he began his studies. I couldn't believe what was happening. It was as if this woman was trying to catch me off-guard. She succeeded. I thought that cameras for the television show Candid Camera must have been nearby; it seemed that she must be joking. Pointing out what we had discussed with her husband and the need for me to know that they were seeing someone to ensure that they, the son, and I were all working together, I reiterated to her what I thought had already been made clear to them both. The parents needed to receive supportive therapy, maybe only four to six sessions, for me to feel comfortable and ethical about getting myself into what could very possibly be a bad situation. It was not fair either to me or to the family to continue treatment when there appeared to be a minefield at home, ready to explode. I didn't want to begin without knowing the terrain and the danger I was getting into. This seemed reasonable. Though my client was probably attempting to reduce his time away from the tennis courts, it was clear from the evidence gathered that there was something awry within the family that could block successful treatment. The vast majority of clients did not say what this boy had said, even if they wanted to avoid punishment or obtain their privileges back.

The mother became upset and defensive. She spoke as her husband had before. My discussion with him did nothing to convince them that something needed to be done. I was very serious about not providing therapy because I didn't want to set Tom or myself up for failure. I was happy to refer them elsewhere if they did not address family dynamics. This was the first time that a family had forced me to take such an action. I felt it unethical to forget what the boy had told me about his father hitting him. Even if it wasn't true, it still signaled a problem within the family. I did not enjoy requiring them to seek treatment because I had to put up with their anger, frustration, and ignorance, but I had learned that at times it was necessary. The family had to realize that a professional believed that the way the family interacted was not productive and would be counterproductive in any attempts to assist this boy who had difficulty with anxiety. Surprising to me, I did not obsess about this case too much. It was so clear to me that I was doing the right thing that any worrying seemed senseless. I felt sorry for this boy and his family. I spoke about the case with my colleagues and that served to reduce my anxiety.

I understood that it would be unpleasant to hear that as a parent you needed to change your behavior in order for treatment to be possible for your son. Change would be difficult, especially during times when your family was being scrutinized. Nevertheless, in general, families need to find the strength and wisdom to make such necessary changes. This is very difficult at best and nearly impossible at worst. To progress with this boy's treatment was the equivalent of a medical doctor helping someone with diabetes while his family was feeding him chocolate every chance they got. No problem exists in a vacuum. The family is very important in influencing, one way or another, how someone responds to treatment of any sort. In this case, the parents never agreed to get help, and they would not participate in treatment. I did not feel that I could continue with the case, and I referred them elsewhere.

Notwithstanding my previous descriptions of these two difficult family cases, I don't want to leave the false impression that all families operate in like manner. The majority of families help treatment along and provide an environment that makes treatment more effective. For these families, what I ask them to do is not easy, either. They have bought into the rationale for CBT and have more hope and confidence in the therapeutic process. Many have read the latest research findings and are aware of the approaches that CBT therapists utilize to maximize behavioral change and symptom reduction. In short, the families that do much of what I request assist their children significantly.

One very important lesson that I have learned while at my current position is that helping everyone is impossible. As other therapists, I sometimes get caught up in believing that I am the only one, the chosen one, that can help a particular client or family. However, some sufferers and their families do not want help. Sure, people want to feel better, but sometimes they are unwilling to behave differently in order that positive change is possible.

Feeling overresponsible for people's welfare the first few years I worked as a therapist, the thought of leaving my job entered my mind. I could not help everyone; perhaps I did not belong in this line of work. Maybe I wasn't cut out for it. I knew on some level that I was performing adequately at my job, but it was hard to see fellow sufferers not receive the help they needed. The first few years were difficult. *I worked so hard to get to this point and now what?*

The anxiety that I experienced those first few years was strong enough for me to take my therapist's suggestion and attend a group where I could receive feedback from others who suffered the scourge of an anxiety disorder. I had never gone to a therapy group led by another therapist and didn't know what to expect. The group met six times on a weekly basis. By the third session, we knew a little bit about each other and felt more comfortable to talk about our "issues."

At the third session, a woman asked, "Would I want to go to a therapist who was not self-assured about his or her abilities and had all these self-doubts swimming in his or her head?" I did not know what to say. Others were also uncertain about what to say. My anxiety soared. I told the group that I was very anxious. The therapist reminded me to allow the feelings to come and go on their own without doing anything ritualistically. Don't reassure myself that everything would work out at my job. In fact, tell myself that maybe things wouldn't work out. Do something that we Westerners are terrible at, to just be. Don't do, just be. By the end of the session, my anxiety had diminished. I also became aware of something extremely important. I was engaging in more mental rituals than I knew about or wanted to admit. After this anxiety-provoking session, I reduced my mental rituals. I stopped fueling the fear that I was incompetent. It turned out that the doubting woman in the group allowed me to learn about my own behavioral responses to anxiety in the group context. Ironically, she helped me by doubting me.

Of course, I eventually came to terms with this fear of being inadequate at work and have usually been able to let it go. It helped to hear from other group members in later sessions that my feelings and the frequency of self-doubting thoughts did not signify genuine incompetence. They empathized with the experience of being bludgeoned by persistent and painful thoughts. I am very grateful that I stayed the course and allowed objective evidence and my understanding of OCD to govern my behavior. I never want anxiety to dictate what I do.

In spite of the lesson learned from the group, I still hated not being able to help someone, whatever the reason was. I know intimately what OCD pain feels like and I wish that there was a magic pill or a magical incantation that could remove all of his or her symptoms. As we know, there isn't. Who knows what the future will bring in regards to treatment? Perhaps an OCD gene will be discovered and treatments will be developed to change the expression of the "anxiety" gene. Despite this uncertainty, I am certain that CBT helps many people and could help many more if they only gave it a chance. Don't give up on it before trying and never let anxiety govern your life.

Chapter 15

EL GRINGO IN PUERTO RICO

Typically, vacations are a time when my OCD improves. The lack of a schedule, responsibilities, and demands is conducive to a more relaxed state of mind. On our first trip to Puerto Rico in the summer of 2001, my wife and I were very fortunate to have great, Spanish-speaking hosts drive us to terrific, exotic destinations. One day, we decided to go to an island off the east coast of Puerto Rico. In order to get to the island, we had to take a ferryboat that left at about 8 A.M. Just to be on the safe side, we estimated that it would take us a good hour and a half to get to the dock. Needless to say, we had to wake up at an ungodly hour, an hour that normal humans are not supposed to ever witness. I think God is telling us something when it's dark.

On the way to the ferry, we came upon a scene that was new to me. A car was completely tipped over on the side of the road and two men were frantically waving their arms attempting to get our attention. They didn't have to gesticulate in the way they did for us to take notice. You couldn't miss the car. I was thinking to myself that I couldn't believe this was happening since we were so close to the departure point for the ferry.

We pulled up alongside this scene and I became very uncomfortable wondering what I should do. What was expected of me at such a moment? My thoughts were racing, but time appeared to slow down. I could see what was happening, but I could not stop it. It was like seeing two trains on a collision course without any possibility of acting to change the inevitable outcome. *Is there a Good Samaritan Law on the books as in the last Seinfeld episode, or is there anything that any of us can do?* The entire time, I was aware that my friend was a medical school student and my wife was a nurse, so I thought that maybe they could assist in some way.

Anyway, I rolled down the window and my friend started speaking Spanish to the man. It turned out that the man wanted help to tip the car back upright so that the police would not become involved. The two men were very drunk and were staggering all over the place. My friend had warned me about the many social problems in Puerto Rico, but I didn't need a close-up view of it.

The entire time we were close to the tipped-over car, I wondered if I should leap out of the car and try to perform first aid on the man. I knew CPR and I was trained in giving first aid. There was some blood; I was very anxious. I didn't know what to do and my friend and wife were just talking to the man. It seemed to me that we should be doing more — that we were wasting time talking. I wasn't saying any of this out loud; it pounded in my mind repetitiously. *I need to do something now because time is running out!* My fear of being responsible for someone else's welfare was coming to the forefront again. My friend told the man that he would call for help at the pier. I had difficulty following the conversation. I was proficient in Spanish, but in situations where people were speaking very fast and my level of anxiety was off the charts, it may as well have been Chinese.

I kept thinking, "There must be something that I can do for this man! There must be something that I can do to help my wife and friend help this man." The entire time my friend was speaking to the man, I felt compelled to open the car door. I'm not sure why, it just felt like the right thing to do. I didn't. Maybe I should have. I began thinking, "I'm in the way of medical people assessing the situation and I'm not really helping . . . and if something really bad happens to the men that it's all my fault. If only I can be selfless and act, not freezing up when I become anxious, those men would be receiving the necessary help that they need." These thoughts, and variations of them, continued to stream into my consciousness, flooding me with thoughts that I reacted to with feelings of extreme guilt, self-pity, and disappointment.

When my friend said that we would call the authorities at the pier, my anxiety initially subsided some. Someone else had taken the bull by the horns and come to a decision about what to do. It was reassuring to me that someone seemed to have the confidence that I was sorely lacking at the time. However, as we continued on to the pier, I could not shake the scary scene of the tipped-over car from my mind. It might as well have been colored and stamped onto my mind. A washable marker wasn't used; it was one of those nasty and hated permanent markers.

While we were waiting at the pier for the boat, there was plenty of time for me to get into a good old-fashioned obsessive state. It didn't help that it was 7:00 A.M. and that I was tired, although I was sure my anxiety would have been high at any time of the day under the same circumstances. I told my wife what my anxieties were and she said that we did all that we could have done and all that anyone would have done back at the crash site. She pointed out that my friend assisted individuals in emergencies all the time at his job, and that he didn't feel it was necessary to do anything more. I felt relieved that the feedback from others ran counter to my feelings. Yet, my anxiety was still there. I told myself to, "Go with the flow" and to "Bring on the anxiety." My admonitions did not change anything. I've noticed that when I get this anxious about an event that actually involves someone (possibly or actually) being hurt, I have to ride it out. I know rationally that I did not hurt or impede others from helping, that OCD was responsible for your feelings. I wanted to refrain from repeating this information in my mind. That action would constitute ritualizing. At that point I knew this, but my feelings were so strong that my view of the chain of events was very foggy and distorted. I kept telling myself that anxiety was not going to hurt me and that it would diminish over time.

While this internal struggle was occurring, what did others observe? They probably saw that I was quieter, less confident, my back stooped over a bit, and my language had become more wavering and uncertain. Decisions were more difficult for me to make and things in the external world were distractions to my self-absorption. I also tended to forget things more, things both significant and insignificant. Typically, the insignificant, less meaningful things were not remembered at all.

We waited at the pier for two or three hours. By the time we stepped onto the boat, my anxiety had decreased significantly, though I still didn't feel as good as I had wanted. The more I thought about the incident after the initial round of questions and images entered my mind, the more confused and foggy I became. It is so, so tempting to try to quickly erase pain away with good, positive, self-reassuring thoughts, but these thoughts were really mental rituals. In this society, everything seems to be at our fingertips and medicine can create all kinds of miracles from growing hair to producing an erection, to providing happiness. We do not do well with patience. Given our technology, we must be able to wipe our minds clean of uncomfortable thoughts and images immediately. This is the seductive trap of OCD. OCD requires us to engage in overanalyzing and performing rituals for its survival. Believe me, I've tried every way in, under, over, through, and around this trap, but none work.

Frequently, we try to eliminate pain and suffering by suppressing thoughts. Increasing the suppression of "bad" thoughts and images adds to the power they possess over us. They must be really, truly bad if we are trying to not think of them. Research strongly supports this assertion. Don't get me wrong. That doesn't mean that you should dwell on "bad" thoughts either (unless you are under the care of a CBT therapist with OCD experience), or attempt to neutralize one thought with another. For example, some people literally think the word good every time they hear the word bad, and think God every time they hear the word devil. These are compulsions and not healthy coping strategies for managing and living with anxiety.

Of course, I wanted the best for the man on the side of the road. However, I did not need to obsess, ritualize, and inhibit anxiety-provoking thoughts to feel as though I did what I could (nothing) in the situation. It was extremely difficult for me to acknowledge that there were limitations imposed on me; I couldn't do everything and was not in control of many things. Sometimes, I can't do anything. I am learning different ways of coping when I feel helpless, vulnerable, and out-of-control. I practice thinking more rationally and I intentionally place myself in difficult situations.

Despite the "drunken men" incident, my OCD generally improved while I was away from the stressors of everyday life, particularly work. When I go on vacation, I become keenly aware of how much stress plays a part in my OCD. However, the disorder does not disappear. In fact, I do not expect my OCD to simply vanish. However, I find myself wishing that it would just disappear and never return. Part of me is still not on vacation. OCD is hovering over me, and I don't care if it does. It's a companion that has the job of challenging my emotional well-being and testing my ability to withstand sudden bursts of anxiety and prolonged anxiety-provoking situations. That's how I see my OCD. It helps me to tolerate the everyday stressors of life and to focus better, and in so doing it makes me stronger. Of course, I don't want OCD and wish I did not have it, but I might as well take something positive from it.

Something that my first psychiatrist once told me has stuck with me to this day. He said, "You didn't ask for OCD." I took that to mean that it was not my fault that I had OCD, therefore it was not helpful to wallow in self-pity and feel really bad for acting and thinking obsessively and compulsively. He was right.

What makes OCD so difficult for me is the intensity, duration, and frequency of my symptoms. The intensity is the variable that is most difficult for others to comprehend. Dr. Rapoport spoke of OCD as "a hiccup of the brain." However, that doesn't address the pain that sufferers experience when they are in the grips of the disorder. I always preferred the "mosquito bite of the mind" metaphor. The more you scratch (compulsion) the itch (obsession), the worse the pain gets. You feel that you can't avoid scratching (performing compulsions). Immediately after a longer episode of scratching is completed, the pain diminishes, but this relief lasts for a very short period of time. The pain resurfaces and becomes more intense than when it started. Likewise, the greater the frequency, duration, and intensity of engaging in compulsive behaviors are, the stronger the OCD becomes and the greater the long-term suffering will be.

Chapter 16

FIGHT OR FRIGHT?

It was Halloween. It was a day that people relished scaring each other and being scared. It had been three months since my trip to Puerto Rico and I had finally recovered from my misadventures. Rather than engaging in any of the traditional activities, I met with one of my clients, an eighteen year-old man who was scared. In Puerto Rico, I felt overly responsible for another's health. My patient, in contrast, did not feel responsible enough for even his own well-being, much less the well-being of others. He was not scared of any costumes or masks, but of living life the way that most of us live it. He was running scared, trying to avoid anxiety, which of course was the same as avoiding life. It is impossible to avoid anxiety or life; eventually realities impinge upon one, always sooner than later. His story was replete with examples of his customary response to stress and anxiety; he took flight rather than fighting the feared stimuli. For my client, every day was filled with Halloween-level fright.

He was so anxious about the prospect of cleaning himself that he believed he really did not know how to wash himself. My client was so terrified of showering that he wanted his family members to help him. Now that's scared and confused! Nothing I have or ever will experience on a Halloween night will ever compare to the fright that this man felt. He was so accustomed to having OCD rules and following them in a rigid, precise manner, and that any deviations from these rules, even ways that were present pre-OCD, did not make any sense to him. He even asked me if he were hospitalized, whether the staff members would shower patients. He needed to break the OCD rules and shower to refresh himself, not to get clean by his OCD standards. In reality, there was no "right" way to shower. Do whatever comes to mind first, allowing your hands to go wherever they do to wash themselves.

Halloween is about quick, rapid bursts of fright such as someone jumping up nearby shouting, "Boo!," suddenly opening a door in front of you, creeping up behind you, or being taken by surprise by your brother as you turn a corner. After the sudden scare, you know immediately that someone is simply trying to scare you and your anxiety dissipates very quickly. OCD anxiety often rapidly peaks, too, and then gradually diminishes over a span of minutes.

Imagine feeling the way you feel when you are extremely scared and experience that feeling pervasively, or at least for a few minutes. That intensity of fear is what OCD sufferers experience on a daily basis, day in and day out. No wonder I see people who do not want to participate in life. Life is too scary! It is so scary that they believe that they gain more by avoiding than by partaking of it, even if the avoiding leaves them in a state of inertia. Inertia is more comfortable to them than moving and fully experiencing life.

When there is such a level of fear and inertia present, the family is that much more important in helping the OCD sufferer to move forward. I believe that on some level, whether they admit it or are aware of it, everyone wants a better life. I work under the assumption that if environmental changes are made, and the contingencies for behaving certain ways are modified, everyone can change in meaningful ways.

Families need to realize that OCD is real, it is painful, and it is a frightening disorder that flares up at inopportune, inconvenient times. Willpower alone does not defeat OCD. Of course, willpower and motivation are important, but willpower does not subdue diabetes, so why should it conquer OCD? I know what you're thinking. You think that OCD is a mental, emotional thing and that such things are controllable; it's all in your head. (Yes, that is the problem.) Yes, frequently we all have certain unacceptable thoughts, feelings, or impulses that we do not act on, indicating that we have a certain level of control. In some cases, we cannot even express them openly. This level of control may be necessary. We better not curse out the boss or say something inappropriate to an attractive person that we see on the street, and we usually don't. We can have much more control over our behavior than over our feelings or thoughts.

OCD is not a logical, rational disorder. Yet, there are kernels of logic entangled in the thought processes of the sufferer. Someone who checks the door or stove repeatedly thinks that a negative consequence can be averted because of the compulsive behavior. Of course, checking something over and over again is not really providing us with any additional information. A common justification (anxiety leads to OCD thinking, which in turn reinforces the OCD behavior) for the compulsive behavior is, "Well, someone could break in and steal things." Or, "The house could catch on fire and a lot of damage could be done." Certainly, if there were a fire, a lot of damage occurs. If someone did break into the house then it would be bad news. The person with OCD equates "could" with "will," "maybe" with "yes," and "there's a one in a million chance" to, "it will definitely happen to me." Instead of taking a leap of faith that all is not as threatening as it appears, the person instead is possessed by doubt, and is ruled by his belief that the likelihood of extremely low-probability disasters are inevitable. The person's flight response activates. (The fight vs. flight response to stress is what I'm referring to here.) Realistically, there is **no** chance of something "bad" or "catastrophic" happening due to an OCD person's thoughts or feelings.

Others have to realize that the individual harassed by OCD may not be able to differentiate between "could" and "would." This is not because of a lack of intelligence, but because this is what OCD does to someone; it is the very essence of OCD. Trying to convince sufferers that they should not perform their rituals is akin to attempting to persuade someone who suffers from depression that sleeping a lot does not help their plight. In both instances, the individual knows this on some level. However, the disorder clouds the mind and the person feels more comfortable with taking the safe way out, gratifying and relieving the individual for the moment, but reinforcing and strengthening OCD in the longer view. In the case of OCD, the safe way equals unhealthy stagnation.

Earlier in my career, I would occasionally get OCD-related doubts at work about the job I did. One evening in particular captures some key descriptive points that are important in understanding OCD and the role of fear and anxiety. I will describe OCD "freezing," "flighting," and "fighting."

It started at the home of a twelve year-old client. I make "house-calls" frequently, meeting the person in an environment that is more likely to provoke high states of anxiety. At the end of the session as I was leaving for my next "in vivo" house-call, I was talking to my client's mother and she asked me how things were going with treatment. After I responded positively to her query, she stated that she had not observed progress. As sometimes happens, a client may make progress before it is obvious to family members. Click! My OCD light-switch turned on immediately after she said "lack of progress." Little did I know that this one OCD light-switch was the start of an epic anxiety journey. This is what normally took place before Halloween-level anxiety surfaced. The situation required that I continue talking with the lady while taking my leave, and the click, or rather my reaction to it, were pushed aside. I thank God everyday for being able to go on even when, on some level, I feel unable to. This is God's gift to me and to the millions of others who struggle in the face of terrible, uncertain, doubtful, insecure, helpless, and incompetent feelings.

Having attempted to leave the house earlier to arrive at another client's house on time, I began my drive frustrated for failing to start my rounds earlier. It seemed that I never had enough time for others or for myself. I realized that my OCD (fear of making mistakes that could possibly lead to horrific consequences) and my perfectionistic tendencies had arrived on the scene. As I drove away, I began to sense that something just wasn't right. The width of the lane of the road appeared to narrow and I couldn't seem to stay between the lines. I was aware of being more vigilant of other cars coming my way. I told myself that this was just my OCD driving my anxiety. Because OCD was what these uncomfortable feelings were all about, I told myself that I was not going to worry about them. I calmed myself down momentarily. However, it was dark and raining and the roads were really narrow and unfamiliar. In fact, I began to think that I was traveling in the wrong direction. Nothing was turning out the way I wanted it to. I couldn't put my finger on what had triggered the heightening of my anxiety.

Of course, when she mentioned that she had not seen any progress in her son, it upset me, even though I had definitely seen improvements during our sessions. I usually mentally cringe when someone says something I don't want to hear, especially something that I might interpret as questioning my ability as a therapist. Pinpointing the trigger or cue for anxious feelings is very helpful and useful to me. The trigger helps explain the reason for my anxiety. Being aware of the connection between the trigger and OCD allows me to be more rational about anxiety-provoking situations. Fortunately, this time, the connection became apparent very quickly, being a fairly obvious one. *This is just my OCD acting up. Since it's just my OCD, it's not anything about which I need to be anxious.* When I think like this, I'm acknowledging the presence of an overreaction that is OCD.

Unfortunately, I began to obsess in earnest about the treatment regimen with the young boy I had left. Obsessing? You ask why it was obsessing? A person with OCD knows the difference between OCD and non-clinical mood states. The difference is expressed in its intensity, frequency, and duration. Basically, it is very hard to shake the thoughts out of my mind. For instance, usually by listening to a favorite song and singing it, I can stop thinking about virtually anything. On the contrary, with an obsession, it doesn't work like that. One becomes a slave to the thought, punished for thinking it and punished for not.

Over and over again, I reflected on what had transpired in my interactions with the boy. *Oh, man! I hate this windy road. Here comes a car. Be careful! Didn't I screw up with this boy? Didn't I just get too close to that car? Didn't I just hear a noise? Oh, that was the radio? Or was it? There aren't any trumpets playing in this song. That sound was too high pitched.* In my mind, thoughts of the present and of the past interwove to form a mixed up, blended, unclear, and obscure whole new version of the present.

Disorientation and confusion ran rampant in my mind. Nonetheless, I did not feel these two emotions quite as intensely as I usually did. I was sure that the Klonopin was helping me through the speed bumps of my life. By means of positive self-statements, I was successful at returning to the realm of rationality. I told myself, "You're doing a fine job. He is definitely making progress. This family is difficult to deal with, and it is hard for non-professionals to understand OCD, so give yourself a break."

Typically, what happens in a situation when an obsession has already begun (fear of making mistakes in treatment that can lead to a loss in someone's well-being) and other anxieties appear (i.e., driving) is that my mind appears cloudy and murky. My mind is stuck on the first anxiety-provoking event, yet something pulls me forward towards the second anxiety-provoking event. Stuck between two points, and not knowing where to go or what to do, I choose which obsession to "handle" (obsess or ritualize about) first. Naturally, going on with life and being with the anxiety, and not performing my rituals when I feel stuck, would be the healthiest course of action. Nevertheless, at that precise moment in time, I sometimes feel compelled to act on my anxiety. Fortunately, humans can normally choose when and how to act. I do not have to retrieve and revisit anxious moments. The choice to act in a healthier way is easier at certain times more than at others. In this example, I forced myself to look ahead, keep my eyes on the road, and think about what I was doing. This time it worked and my obsessions and anxiety faded.

Nearing my next client's house, anxiety mounted again. I was very late and was embarrassed for showing up forty-five minutes late. The traffic on the major highway was stop-and-go, moving at a crawl most of the way. Merging into a left lane from an entrance ramp led to a nervous reaction on my part. *Again, this damn driving anxiety.* Part of me felt like looking back to make sure that I had not caused an accident, and the other part was telling myself to look at the road ahead and live through the anxiety. The tension between backwards vs. forwards, and past vs. present is omnipresent in my relationship to my OCD thoughts and feelings.

Oh, no! My client just peered out the window and saw me approaching the house. I felt like such an idiot. *I am an idiot. Wait a minute! Remember, the traffic was awful.* Everybody on the Beltway was late in arriving to his or her destination. At any rate, I would have been thirty minutes late even if I had left my first client's house on time. I wondered what would happen if I just drove away. *Oh, this is ridiculous. They will understand. They live near the highway and have assuredly arrived late to places themselves. What else am I supposed to do? I have to face them and tell them what happened even though it is going to be very hard to do.*

I knocked on the door and my client's mother quickly answered. While I apologized for being so late, she jokingly pretended to hit me over the head. I still felt a little rattled by all the anxieties. Suddenly, surprisingly, two of my client's friends came walking into the living room with my client while I was talking to the mother. She was reporting how poorly her son had done the previous week. I maintain confidentiality when talking to my clients and their parents. I felt awkward and anxious speaking in front of his friends, but they were there and I had to at least say "hi" to my client.

I get very anxious regarding confidentiality and privacy. One of the mantras that I learned as a graduate student was, "Never breach a client's confidentiality." Being a world-class Olympic champion in catastrophic thinking, my initial knee-jerk reaction that resulted from this uncomfortable situation was thinking about worst-case scenarios. Images of dramatic court cases involving Machiavellian attorneys who grill me for every sordid detail about my night at my client's door raced through my mind. Upon recognizing such absurd and silly thinking, I laughed to myself. I was surprised that at the graduation ceremonies they didn't tattoo a dictum about confidentiality on my body, but that would not be a nice social work thing to do. Could you imagine the headline, "Crazed social workers caught tattooing in public?" Anyway, you get the point that it was extremely important in the code of ethics of my profession. Anything resembling breaking confidentiality led me to experience anxiety.

My anxiety and discomfort was appropriate and adaptive in this case, because his mother and his friends were invading the space between my client and me, his therapist. Making "house-calls" can lead to problems with space; sometimes it is difficult to get an inviolable area in which to speak. The worst part about the whole scenario was that there did not seem to be any way out. I was penned in. I could not turn around and walk out the door to escape my discomfort because it was my job to talk to the boy and to cope with the mother's poor assessment of her son's condition. As I stood at the door, I felt Halloween-level anxiety because I had to be and work in a very personally vulnerable place. The four obsessions from the previous house, the road, and where I was standing converged to cause me great discomfort.

There wasn't any time to insert any concerns regarding privacy. Looking around the room, it did not seem that anyone at the house cared if I said, "Hello" or made some profound interpretation about my client's social tendencies. Perhaps I could have told an off-color joke and no one probably would have taken offense, figuring that it must be a new therapeutic technique developed for this kind of awkward situation. It would be something to break the ice. Such openness with a group of strangers sharing potentially very personal information did not sit right with me. However, no "inside" information was exposed and I kept my comments very general and impersonal. Of course, the individuals were not strangers to the family, but rather my client's friends. Even so, they had no right to know anything about my client and our therapeutic relationship.

Later, reflecting back on what had transpired, I concluded that I was more worried about making a mistake than I was about what actually happened in the situation. I was hypervigilant about exactly what my client and I said. All focus went to the words and our facial and body gestures. I was protecting myself from experiencing more anxiety; I did not want more. Later in the evening, time and distance provided me an enhanced capacity to really see the "what," "why," "how," "now what," and "so what" of my behavior.

While walking back to the car after the session, I felt a great sense of relief that the episode was over, maybe not in my head but at least at their house. Being by myself, my guard was down and I felt confused and mixed-up. I always experience this after living through several anxiety-provoking situations in a relatively short period of time. The best example I can give to describe the feeling is to imagine several radios simultaneously playing a different favorite song and each vying for your attention. You feel compelled to listen to one and focus exclusively on it to fully enjoy it, but when you attempt that course of action, the other songs interrupt the process. You simply cannot get satisfaction from two at the same time because you can't pay full attention to each of them. I have learned that the most helpful thing to do is to try not to listen to only one song at a time, but rather to say to myself, "Go with the flow." Listen to whatever pops into my head, even if it's jumbled. Live with the anxiety, observe it, experience it, and feel it without judging my internal experiences.

By this time, I was driving in mental and physical cruise control. This is what normally happened after a Halloween-level anxiety episode. Internally, everything was coming at me at once, and in trying to make sense of it all, I was coming up with nothing clear and distinct. It's akin to mental over-stimulation. When one is over-stimulated internally or externally, the natural response is to first escape the area, and then arrive at a new calmer equilibrium. Obsessive, internally-focused people can become tired of this over-stimulation. They are very acutely aware of any change in speed, intensity, and duration of their running thoughts. Driving all this chaos was my old buddy "anxiety."

Individuals who suffer from OCD do have difficulty "letting go" of their thoughts, behaviors, and habits. In addition, they suffer from difficulties of "picking up." What this means is that some sufferers regularly struggle to get going, get moving, and get started doing something. They shy away from doing something (e.g. showering, making a decision) because of a tremendous fear of the perceived negative consequences that will ensue if they do take action. Many people with OCD start an action (showering) and have difficulty stopping the action. Others don't begin in the first place because they realize that once they get into the shower they cannot live up to their own internal expectations of being clean. They will still feel dirty, and they know this. It seems easier for them to not confront the feared stimulus (shower) in the first place, so they don't. When I ask people to take a shower in five minutes, they look at me incredulously. They ask, "How can you get clean in five minutes? Why get into the shower if I'm not even going to complete it?" It's as if they believe that they are cleaner by not showering than if they did venture into the shower for only a short period of time.

Sufferers' responses to perceived dangers vary, a sign of the struggle of "letting go." Some tend to avoid, escape, and take flight from certain stimuli, events, and environmental cues. Others frequently remain to fight in the anxiety-provoking environment, some are prone, despite attacking the OCD, to engage in some compulsions to keep the anxiety down so that they feel more "settled and focused." Others who choose to fight stand up to the OCD and weaken it, not performing any rituals. The third group might "freeze" if they are involuntarily forced or become acutely aware of higher-than-expected levels of anxiety. Members of this group might experience a "purgatory" or "pause" phenomenon on account of being left to make up their minds if they want to fight or flight. Maybe they cannot "keep up" with the mental chatter. Clearly, some individuals in the second group are using E/RP and weakening their OCD. The first group is in flight and is strengthening their OCD. The third group consists of people who do the most common, convenient thing; they "freeze." They carry on with life, but also carry around OCD. They fight it when they can and feel like it, and flight when the anxiety elevates too highly.

Unfortunately, the third group consists of people who sometimes literally "freeze" (remain motionless) by ceasing all activity for varying lengths of time, waiting for a ritual from themselves or others. Group members' actions stop for seconds or minutes at a time; their inaction is very conspicuous to others. At my absolute worst, my actions become more abrupt and less fluid. No one notices the difference, but I feel it. I might pause momentarily and imperceptibly for a split-second, trying to "catch up" processing all incoming information. My compulsive internal self attempts to get back in-sync with my external self. It is very clear to me that I am having a problem with mental processing. The world is coming at me at one hundred miles per hour, but my mind can only realistically keep up with cognitive and sensorial input traveling at thirty miles per hour. In these moments, I try to think and experience more than I feel comfortable with, flooding my mind with random, fragmented pieces of internal experiences. It takes practice to "just be" and tolerate this vexing whirlwind. Focus on the present and observe what is transpiring without judging or criticizing.

This book aims to help people become members of the second group. Fighting scary and terrifying stimuli and confronting discomfort head-on without using rituals is the best way to live with OCD.

Chapter 17

THE THERAPIST WHO STOLE CHRISTMAS

My personal and professional experience with the "freeze" phenomenon helped me immensely in the case that will be discussed in this chapter. The sufferer represents one whom is paralyzed and incapacitated by elevated anxiety, profound slowness, and wavering indecision. Instead of fighting, flighting, or freezing for a short time, Holly's obsessive-compulsive slowness was a constant and persistent trait. In effect, she was perpetually frozen, at least to some degree.

It was December 11 in the year 2001. The Christmas season, along with Hanukkah and Kwanzaa, were in high gear. We all know that this time of year places additional demands upon us that are not present at any other time of the year, at least not in regards to number and compactness of events over time. Many people do get stressed out and feel physically and emotionally exhausted. Some try to do too many things in a short span of time.

If anyone exemplified dread and a lack of preparedness for the upcoming holiday season, it was Holly. She liked and appreciated the holidays just like anyone else, but the holidays represented one huge deadline for her -- a deadline that would not be moved for any reason. Christmas occurs on the 25th whether we want it to or not. It is not on the 23rd, 24th, 26th, 27th, or any other date for that matter. Christmas will always occur on the 25th, no matter what. If someone celebrates it on the 26th, it just doesn't feel the same. It's not Christmas any more. It has already passed.

Holly abhorred deadlines. Why? Because the very definition of the word deadline means "the latest time by which something must be done or completed." The word "must" was the difficult word to swallow for Holly. It didn't state "may," could," might," or "would." "Must" denoted that a commitment had been made and, more importantly, action had to take place. Initiation of action was hard for Holly, particularly when such a fixed deadline loomed on the horizon. Sure, she could miss a barber appointment, doctor appointment (non-emergency), shopping outing, or various additional errands, and the consequences did not appear so severe. She could reschedule or have someone else perform the tasks she did not do, but nobody was going to reschedule Christmas.

I identified with Holly's battle with procrastination and its typical partner in crime, perfectionism. Holly belonged on a point near procrastination at the far end of a timeliness-procrastination continuum. I was much closer to the normal range, but I have had my share of problems over the years. For example, during graduate school, I had a penchant for waiting until the last minute to turn in a paper. I arrived two and one-half hours **after** a class to turn in a paper due that class period. Fortunately, I found my professor walking outside and handed the paper to him. It was so embarrassing to see him give me a quizzical, incredulous look that said, "Why are you giving this to me now?"

While finishing the assignment, my anxiety soared as I typed the last few words. I fought with the printer to get the paper to look respectable. The specifications never seemed to be correct; I couldn't get the spacing right and the entire text would print on the far right side of the paper. It was an older printer and there were frequent problems with the paper feeding straight into it. I frantically attempted to complete everything. Like Holly, my anxiety increased in proportion to the time remaining before the deadline. Unlike Holly, whose anxiety started to rise weeks, even months before a deadline, my anxiety began only hours before time expired. Thankfully, I was able to cope with the briefer period of anticipatory anxiety. Poor Holly, she did not have much of a chance, without professional assistance, to start or complete a task.

I was not a person who thrived in high-pressure situations. I needed to give myself extra time to allow for the unexpected and begin working earlier. Breaking the assignment into small, manageable chunks and starting earlier were incompatible tasks with putting things off. I experienced enough anxiety. I did not need to engage in self-defeating behavior unnecessarily. Becoming aware of my limits and giving myself sufficient time to complete a project were very important, especially since I had an anxiety disorder.

On the other hand, Holly gave herself excessive time to complete a task; however, she never got around to it. She was very perfectionistic. The inside of the house had to be impeccably decorated. She had such a wearisome time engaging in goal-directed behavior. Her aesthetic tastes for the elegant, spotless, and the extra-added niceties frustrated her more because she felt unable to complete the tasks she so much desired to finish. She didn't feel prepared to move on to the next phase of a project, or, for that matter, to begin it. Everything must be checked, rechecked, and checked again. Forgetting something and doing things contrary to her preferred, particular, and idiosyncratic sequence validated her sense that she had to continue to ponder the task before acting. Naturally, everyone forgets something from time to time, and fortunately it normally doesn't result in any severe consequences.

Just the fact that she forgot was an indication to Holly that she needed to slow down, take it easy, and even avoid actions. Not remembering something was very anxiety-provoking and signaled to her to stop, slow down, and take it easy.

Again, OCD, and its frequent companion perfectionism, got in the way of healthy functioning. Swimming against the flow was what treatment dictated. Treatment for Holly consisted of ascertaining what the rules of her behavior were and encouraging her to do the opposite. For example, she liked to put up scores of snowmen decorations inside the house. I suggested that she behave differently so that her thoughts and feelings would change and help her grow and leave the rut in which she found herself. Put up less! I requested that she put up fewer decorations and she looked at me panic-stricken. It seemed that I had told her that one of her relatives had just died. She was shocked because in her mind Christmas was not Christmas without every one of her snowmen in her collection prominently displayed in her residence. This was also the way it was in years past, and therefore it was mandated (in her belief system) that it had to be the way that the house would be spruced up this year. She said, "No, not that. I won't put up even one less snowman." So we agreed that she would decrease the number of other trinkets and extras that she wanted to place around the house.

It was now December 21. Holly and I had agreed that by December 19, the house would be completely finished. We made this deadline December 16, leaving her plenty of time to work on the house. If the house was not finished by the therapy session on December 19, we would work on it during our time together. Each decoration that was left undisturbed after I left her house on December 19 represented a victory for health and growth. Alternatively, each decoration that she moved represented a victory for OCD, perfectionism, and procrastination.

Unexpectedly, Holly had finished a good portion of the decorating. All that was left undone was placing decorations on the windowsill. The remaining decorations were next to the windows ready to go on immediately. All accomplished steps, no matter how small, were signs of health and an indication of flexibility, improved decision-making, and most importantly, action.

During the session, I acted as a distracter, encourager, and counter. I spoke to her continuously and wanted her to talk to me while working, doing two things at once. Simultaneous actions functioned to heighten anxiety and to disallow her to engage in mental checking and analyzing. If she slowed down, I would start counting to five. She knew that this was her cue to make a decision rapidly, but I only had to do this three times in one and one-half hours.

I kept telling her to place the decoration on the first available place she saw. Her tendency was to search for the "perfect" spot to place each decoration. Each one had to be so far away from the next, a red one couldn't be near another red one, and each type of decoration had to be at a certain distance from its same kind. She turned an enjoyable, pleasurable task into a rigid, rule-based, unsatisfying one.

She was afraid that she would become very sloppy, spontaneous, and careless if she gradually shaped her behavior to mimic that of relaxed, casual people. I told her that I was not trying to change her underlying personality. I was only trying to smooth the rough edges and assist her to participate much more fully in life. In stating this, I was attempting to break the defenses she had constructed against change and make treatment more non-threatening. Nevertheless, some of her basic assumptions about behavior did need a little changing in order for treatment to be efficacious. I speak more about an underlying personality disorder in the chapter titled "Setting Yourself Up For Failure."

In treatment in general, we targeted certain, specific behaviors that were acting as "OC"stacles. Of course, adorning the windowsills was not one of the more important targeted behaviors on our behavioral change list. The successful completion of this task did not signify functioning at its highest level, and was not meeting one of life's essential needs. Christmas came only once a year, yet her ability to demonstrate increased speed and flexibility with the ornaments increased the likelihood that she would be much more likely to behave in the same manner in daily aspects of her life. Examples of these included showering, grooming, caring for her hygiene, getting dressed, and leaving the house before she felt ready. Fortunately, once her Christmas behaviors improved, she made some progress in these more important areas as well.

Another targeted Christmas behavior for Holly's treatment occurred when she and her mother went to the tree farm to cut down their Christmas tree. Her mother needed to provide her with a reasonable amount of time to choose a tree (twenty minutes). If she was unable to pick one within that time frame, the mother was to select the tree. This was not being mean. This was a therapeutic step that would help her learn to make decisions in a timely manner. If she wanted to choose the tree, she couldn't walk around the tree farm for two hours until she found the tree that fit her idea of a suitable Christmas tree. Her family couldn't accommodate her in this fashion. It was not fair to anyone. I was hopeful about the tree since Holly responded well to quick counts up to five or ten to make quicker decisions with decorations in the house.

Eventually, Holly realized that to enjoy the holiday she would need to lighten up. Is it better to assure yourself that you will completely and utterly relish one percent of Christmas or "only" experience a moderate amount of pleasure from ninety-nine percent of the holiday? It is curious and sad that people sometimes choose the former.

I had never met anyone like Holly, except for Wayne. I knew Wayne one year earlier, and there were many similarities in the two cases. I was socialized to believe that men did not worry and fuss about appearances, at least not as much as him. "Real men" did not care if there was one less decoration. They did not spend that much time and use so many products in the bathroom!! Women could worry and obsess about their hair, nails, and other such matters. On the contrary, men did not have this luxury. Maybe my value and belief systems slanted towards the rigid Neanderthal view that work, play, hygiene, interior decorating, and other tasks and activities of life consisted of a man's way to do things, and a woman's way to do things. Or perhaps Wayne really was gay. I didn't possess any proof for this speculation, but I had wondered. Realizing that his OCD greatly prolonged the time he spent engaging in "appearance" behaviors, I rationalized and intellectualized that his behavior was a consequence of his OCD. On the other hand, OCD did not make him care as much as he did.

I questioned Wayne's sexuality more than most guys, not only because of my socialization, but also because I still sporadically obsessed about whether I was gay or others thought that I was gay. After I left his house, I felt uneasy and unsettled. Through self-reflection, therapy, and the processing of each therapy session with Wayne, I had learned that the probability was high for me to interpret any perceived "out of bounds" (anything resembling effeminate behavior) behavior to mean that someone was homosexual. My OCD rendered Wayne's case extremely challenging. I became anxious whenever I was near him. Occasionally, I doubted my sexual orientation. His and my behavior were put under a microscope and thoroughly examined. I misinterpreted some of his and some of my behaviors.

Wayne's behavior required another perspective, one that would take all that I had learned and apply it in order for me to see anew. This was a difficult task due to my rigid thought system about gender roles. However, I was able to continue to work effectively with Wayne because I did challenge some of my unreasonable, irrational, and outdated beliefs and make the necessary changes. It didn't matter to me morally or ethically if he was gay. Just because he appreciated the aesthetic, stylish, and refined did not necessarily indicate that a man was gay. In comparison, my anxiety did not connote that I was gay, either.

Freezing is a common phenomenon that has not received the attention that it deserves. I have provided some examples of the experience that many people go through. OCD sufferers frequently use flighting (avoidance) and freezing to separate themselves from their anxiety.

Chapter 18

STIGMA, INSURANCE,
AND YOUR MENTAL HEALTH

I was running late to a session and feeling anxious about it, yet my client didn't say anything to me about being late. In spite of my trepidation, his mother only mentioned the predicament that she had encountered attempting to recover some of the money spent on psychotherapy from the insurance company. During the session, thankfully, I was able to turn off a continuing stream of self-critical, self-doubting statements about my tardiness and focus on the task at hand. The session went well.

I traveled to the next person's house and took the time to muse about the advantages and resources that most of my clients and their families possessed. Many families were affluent and paid out-of-pocket for services rendered, opting not to interface with the insurance companies due to a low return rate, or because they were concerned about the privacy and confidentiality aspects of dealing with a third party. I could not fathom having enough money to pay out-of-pocket. Since it was a forty-five minute jaunt to my next client's house, I also pondered the state of insurance coverage for mental health, and society's stigma regarding emotional disturbances. Parity did not exist for mental health coverage in part because of the prejudice and discrimination sufferer's experience. I will elaborate upon my experiences working at an insurance company later in the chapter.

There were many pitfalls and obstacles to treatment for myself and others because of misunderstandings, realities, and biased thinking. First, I wished that CBT was more accessible to the average person. Many individuals did not attempt CBT for one or more of the same reasons that kept me from doing so. As a teenager and young adult, my family and I, as many middle-class families in our society, did not have the resources for full CBT treatment. Second, my psychiatrists did not refer me to a CBT practitioner. Third, I believed (as others did) that CBT could not help me with my OCD since I was an obsessive individual and not someone who washed his hands or checked stoves or doors. (I have come to learn that almost everyone has compulsions, they come sometimes in the covert, cognitive variety.) Lastly, many sufferers believed that CBT was akin to a mild form of torture, and that perception intimidated and scared people away from trying CBT. I heard this belief many times at the support group I led.

Cost and time were sometimes prohibitive factors for treatment. The assessment phase of treatment takes between five and ten hours. Most sufferers come for treatment one time each week for a one hour session. There are three factors that lead a therapist to strongly consider meeting more frequently each week and having longer sessions. The three indicators that intensive therapy may be more efficacious are: the presence of severe symptomatology and/or functional impairment and/or severe distress; the knowledge that weekly therapy (sometimes despite the client's completion of CBT exercises outside of the office) is insufficient for expected symptom reduction; and the desire (in moderate to severe cases) to experience moderate to marked symptom reduction at a more rapid pace. For example, college students only have a small block of "free" time in the summer to participate intensively in therapy.

In an intensive, each session is typically two hours. An intensive lasts two to five days a week for two or three weeks. Subsequent to the intensive phase, the sufferer still needs to be seen to maintain gains made in the intensive phase and to make further gains if necessary and desired. At approximately one hundred and fifty dollars per hour, this is a very costly endeavor and, at times, a prohibitive one. Treatment is very expensive and typically costs three to five thousand dollars; the total cost depends on the severity of symptoms, the response to treatment, and the time the client spends practicing exposures outside of the office.

Another possible "OC"stacle to good treatment is insurance coverage. It is terrible for all types of mental health treatment. Physical anomalies are covered well, but the mental (emotional) health of the patient is sometimes sadly neglected. There is so much discrimination and so many people with emotional disorders; it seems the people suffering and their friends and family members need to pull together and stake their claim to parity in insurance coverage. With tens of millions of people suffering from emotional disturbances, sheer numbers can force the industry's hand. There are six to nine million OCD sufferers alone. Fortunately, some in Congress are currently trying to pass legislation that provides parity in coverage for mental health disorders. There is hope that coverage will improve.

It is also the case that a large number of people who complain of certain physical symptoms (headaches, ulcers, blood pressure, and even heart problems) can also be assisted by improved mental health coverage. In fact, many physical maladies can be prevented if mental health coverage improves and sufferers take advantage of available mental health services. Insurance companies will save money by focusing more on physical symptoms that are frequently psychogenic. The mental, physical, and spiritual components of our being are intertwined into one whole. The mental is the physical and the physical is the mental. I suppose that parity is not a politically powerful enough cause yet, but it will be. It is only right and just that it should be.

I had a personal experience in early 2002 that smacked of discrimination against recipients of mental healthcare. Unbeknownst to me, I needed to receive my medication from a mail pharmacy. I had not been informed about the change. I had my psychiatrist send the company a fax with all the required information. To make sure that I was going to get my medication quickly, I sent a written prescription to my insurance company, too. Nothing happened for a few days. I called the company eight times to inquire about the status of the Prozac. I had none left and was beginning to feel mildly depressed. I kept getting the run around. I told several different employees that I had no medication left and that my doctor had faxed the required information. Each person said that it had not been processed yet, even though I had received two calls telling me that it had been. I definitely started to feel as though they were not taking my condition seriously. All that had to be done was for the company to call my doctor and tell him that no medication was on the way. Although my depression deepened and I had made them aware of this fact, it had not spurred any further action. I wondered what would have happened if I had had a problem with a prescription for a blood pressure or a cholesterol medication. Would I have received my medication in a timely manner without any hassles? Sadly, I think that I would have received medication for a "physical" ailment. I finally received my medication after ten days of the run-around with the insurance company.

One month after the medication fiasco, this entire issue of stigma was brought up by a client's mother. She was livid (appropriately so) that her daughter's OCD and Tourette's Disorder (TD) were not covered by insurance as other "physical" problems were. I say "physical" problems because both OCD and TD are at least partially a result of biochemistry. Afflictions that are deemed physical (heart, diabetes, respiratory, etc.) by the insurance companies are covered at a greater rate, sometimes at a significantly higher rate. Emotional disturbances like OCD and TD, even though current research clearly demonstrates a biochemical link, are not covered as "physical" problems are. It doesn't make sense, and it is totally unjust and discriminatory to handle OCD, TD, and many other emotional problems differently.

Somehow, people see an emotional problem as a weakness, as something to be hidden and kept secret from the rest of society. Members of society think that the sufferer diagnosed with an emotional disorder can't cope with whatever life situations he or she faces. Because of their laziness or their inability to improve their lot, the naysayers say, "Why should we pay for a problem that the person can do something about? They have control over their lives."

The difference between OCD and diabetes, for example, is that people can observe and understand the reasons and consequences of suffering from diabetes, but some can't see and are not willing at times to educate themselves about emotional disturbances. "Why not?," you ask. First, society doesn't reward people who talk about their emotional problems. People don't want to hear about them and easily dismiss both the individual and the problem. Some say that these difficulties are not going to get you where you want to go in life. Second, why should you talk about such negative issues? Some individuals who suffer emotionally are afraid to find out more about themselves and their friends and families in therapy, rationalizing that there may be something painful dug up, or that they will feel confused and incomplete after all the pieces of their lives are not put back together again. Third, some people have a real fear about even being near or associated with someone who has a condition that they neither have nor comprehend. Maybe they are a little obsessive-compulsive (who isn't?) about remaining distant from mental health issues, and they do not want to learn any more about the subject.

I reacted similarly to the stigma of OCD. A decade ago, I was completely and utterly scared out of my mind to even think about revealing any information about my OCD. Boy, have times changed. It's probably because I'm surrounded by OCD for much of the day. I often treat sufferers at work and sometimes experience OCD during my off times.

I'm sure that when this book gets published I will be concerned about what my family, friends, colleagues, and others think about me. This is a very revealing and personal book; I don't hold back in telling my story. I'm determined not to mull over or dwell on it. Moreover, I have already practiced not obsessing about what others think. While writing this book, my mother-in-law and her husband both discovered that mental illness is a part of my life. They have both been extremely supportive of my endeavor and have not treated me any differently after I told them about my diagnosis.

The stigma of mental disorders is a real problem. Unfortunately, this society believes that everyone should "pull themselves up by their bootstraps" and "will it away." People should deny and shake free of an emotional problem all by themselves. There may be more self-help books written today and more press about different emotional disturbances; however, mental illness is not a subject that comes up in conversation. It is treated with a "Hush, hush." If it is talked about, it is usually not with the sensitivity and respect that it deserves. There will continue to be a stigma until people are not so afraid of opening up.

Mental illness is a well-guarded secret, protected with all the forces that the family can marshal. On the other hand, sometimes it is a loud and annoying statement. A statement that suggests that someone is benefiting from its existence in some distorted way. It can pull families together or rip them apart more effectively than a machete. In short, mental illness is a very powerful force on the landscape of human experience and functioning. It is scary and hard to comprehend for the general population; therefore, a strong stigma is maintained.

I agree that the state of one's mental health is not everyone's business, and that large corporations and other individuals should not have access to this information if that is the sufferer's choice. However, I also believe that denial, minimalization, rationalization, shame, guilt, and anxiety for behaving in a certain manner are only strengthening the very same chains that are holding all our fellow sufferers captive. Part and parcel of OCD is the secrecy, anxiety, and inhibition that pervade most sufferers' relationships with others. Thus, the very nature of OCD contributes to its perceived relatively low rate of frequency. However, we know that there are millions of individuals in this country alone who know the pain. Everyone reading this knows at least one acquaintance who experiences OCD symptoms, and likely knows somebody diagnosed with the disorder.

Why don't people at churches speak about emotional disorders during the prayer time as they do about physical problems? Why do families lie about why their family member died? Why does a family not take the advice of a professional who is well acquainted with a certain disorder? Why do individuals and families stay stuck in a seemingly never-ending unhealthy pattern even when they are unhappy about their current situation? Why don't I talk about my OCD with my colleagues or any of my friends? Why do people get fired because they suffer from a disorder? Why do people's insurance plans not pay for OCD and other mental disorders at the same rate as heart disease? Why aren't there OCD walks and runs as there are for sufferers of other health problems? The questions go on and on; the answers tell us a lot about the stigma of emotional disorders.

My dream is that some day we will look differently at individuals with all types of mental disorders and treat them with the respect and dignity that they deserve. The rights of women, blacks, and homosexuals have been examined and movements have won some well-deserved freedoms (but not enough) -- freedoms that the rest of us take for granted. Only recently was there anything that could be called a national call to helping people with disabilities. The Americans with Disabilities Act (ADA) of 1990 was the first step, providing more opportunities for individuals who require some accommodations at the job in order to be a productive and contributing citizen. Of course, this is just the first step. Most people with OCD are not disabled, at least not because of the OCD alone. Many people are suffering silently around you, people who are sometimes living a life of quiet desperation. They can frequently do what they have to do, but pleasure and enjoyment are sucked out of their lives, leaving them numbly battling an unseen, incessant force.

Although I am complaining about the lack of societal communication and education about OCD and other emotional disorders, I am often amazed at how open and candid people are about their disorders in therapy sessions. This talkative group includes children and adolescents. People want to be helped so badly that they are willing to speak about very embarrassing topics and risk being ridiculed and deprecated. For instance, people discuss very unusual acts they perform in order to ensure themselves that their anus is entirely empty and "clean." They talk about esoteric "girlie" magazines that they collect and hoard. They talk about the horrors of masturbation and the fear they have of displeasing God. Incredible stuff. Real stuff that people talk to a therapist about, someone who they don't know on a personal level. Yet familial, interfamilial, or any other interpersonal communication may be shut down by a fear of being found out, a fear of others looking at them oddly, and perhaps fear (maybe even real) of being shunned and ostracized by others.

We can continue to keep mental illness a secret and choose to hear about the crazy acts of a very few people who (like the two sniper suspects who killed at least a dozen people in the Washington, D.C. area in the fall of 2002) symbolize what mental illness is. Or we can look around at our immediate friends and family, acquaintances and colleagues and realize that mental disorders are everywhere, often right in front of us. Anybody, given the convergence of a few factors, can become afflicted with a mental disorder.

I'm not recommending a "coming out" party for all emotionally disturbed individuals, only a dialogue between friends and family. Prayer offered up for a depressed person; the truth about why a person hasn't been at work for a month (and understanding by management on the other end); and the ability to speak to others about something that is distressing and not having to fear retribution are examples of everyday activities when mental illness could be brought up.

We all have our problems and emotional baggage, things that we regret, and bad times when we thought our world had been shattered. This is part of what it means to be fully alive and human. Life is not all a bed of roses. All of us are somewhat obsessive about certain things and compulsive about others. Why can't everyone have a dialogue about problems when we all have them to some degree?

The most egregious example of stigma and discrimination that I have ever experienced occurred when I applied for disability insurance. My wife and I had recently decided to hire a financial planner and one recommendation that he made was to protect ourselves in case one of us could not work. I had never been hospitalized for emotional difficulties and had always worked since the age of seventeen. So I did not think for one minute that I was a high risk to incur a disability. In fact, I didn't believe that I was a risk at all.

My wife is a nurse on a critical care unit. Nurses frequently have chronic back problems. One task that places much stress on her back is turning a patient. The patient can develop bedsores if he or she is not properly managed, and turning needs to be done every two hours. Some of the patients are very obese; it might take four or five nurses to turn a patient. My wife physically exerts herself sometimes for twelve hours a shift. During many shifts, she doesn't get one break in twelve hours. Nurses often develop problems with their lower extremities, especially if they are large themselves. The toll on all nurses' legs and feet is immense considering that they do not get much time to sit. Furthermore, the emotional toll of working with people on the verge of death, and seeing many of them die despite your best efforts, is enormous. My wife is at a relatively high risk of needing disability help somewhere down the line. It is well-known that the percentage of nurses on disability is high compared to other types of employment. In contrast, I, on the other hand, talk to friendly people in my office sitting on a soft, cushy chair.

Physically, I'm under no duress.   My work can be emotionally draining, but not disability-inducing.

Well, I bet that you have guessed, in spite of everything said above, who received disability insurance? That's right. My wife was approved, but I was denied coverage! This was unbelievable! There was not a clearer and more repugnant example of stigma and discrimination anywhere!

Another insurance industry assists to maintain negative views of mental disorders: the health insurance industry. Mental health coverage is abysmal. It is awful because insurance companies can save money by not approving mental health care. They seem to think that mental health is a matter of willpower and not worthwhile of effective treatment. People might need a few sessions to discuss something, but twenty sessions is enough time to discover Atlantis. At least this is how they operate. The individual receiving mental health care has to get better soon. Companies claim that they have to remain solvent, therefore they have to use caution when approving any coverage for any type of problem. They say they can't approve everything. No, they can't. However, there must be parity for mental health coverage. The public would riot in the streets if the care for their diabetes or heart problems was not authorized.

Insurance companies have much information concerning your well-being (or lack thereof) and share it, maybe without your knowledge. Several years ago, I left my job as a psychotherapist and went to work for a company that managed several types of mental health insurance policies in Arizona and New Mexico. My job title was Care Manager. I changed jobs because I wanted to secure employment where I would be earning a fixed salary. My pay as a therapist varied depending upon how many clients I saw that week. I had young children and desired to know exactly what I would be making so we could make a family budget.

As a Care Manager, emergency room doctors or private practitioners called and reported that one of their patients required either inpatient or partial hospitalization for mental health or substance abuse diagnoses. In order for my company to make a decision whether to pay for (authorize) or deny treatment, the professional who called had to answer a plethora of questions, sometimes taking twenty minutes. The questions aimed at acquiring every conceivable piece of information that somebody could know about another's current health and their history of health problems. After the lengthy inquiry, I called one of our psychiatrists (who never actually observed the patient) and told him or her some of the data that I collected, and that person made the decision. I called the psychiatrist if I could not authorize coverage because people did not meet medical criteria. And the criteria were very stringent and supervisors looked over my shoulder sometimes, making sure that I was not approving too much.

(Thank God, I could not deny coverage. My "overresponsible" OCD would have blasted off and traveled into deep space. The difficult part was telling others that the psychiatrist denied treatment. I felt awful when I thought that treatment was indeed necessary and even vital.)

Some of our doctors were occupied at times with other matters and sometimes doctors on the requesting end got very angry when they realized that the approval process was so drawn-out and extensive. One doctor yelled at me and asserted that my company and I were doing a huge disservice to people who needed immediate assistance, not up to two hours later when the decision was rendered. Utilization management staff and others filling the requesting role patiently provided the requisite information since they were savvy with the process. They learned how to massage the answers to reflect their beliefs concerning the patient's needs. On my end, though twenty minutes of questions accumulated much data about the patient, our doctor's did not seek much information to deny or approve coverage. At the core, patients had to have ideas of suicide or homicide, a plan of execution, and intent to kill themselves or others to be approved for inpatient hospitalization. In other words, it was rather difficult to get someone help because it took meeting extreme criteria in order that the patient's behavior necessitated intervention. It took a short period of time to make a very important decision.

It was a very fast-paced, anxiety-inducing work environment. As a general rule, I worked more productively when I could go at my own pace. I was extremely anxious and self-conscious when I worked for the insurance company. Somebody was always looking over my shoulder, sometimes literally. I trembled as never before due to my very high anxiety levels. When I did eat lunch, I shook uncontrollably and expended much energy trying to conceal this behavior. I felt awful, my head fogged up, and I did not know what to do first. I was afraid of making a mistake because my supervisors had yelled at me three or four times. A mistake at this job could still negatively affect somebody's life. Maybe somebody wouldn't get the treatment they required because I typed and relayed the information inaccurately and incorrectly to the psychiatrist. Perhaps, I did not present a strong enough case. Or perhaps I should have authorized more care even though the medical necessity criteria for that level of care were dubiously met.

Paperwork became the focus of my anxieties as it had at my psychotherapy position. Contrary to my belief entering the position, forms and documents complicated my emotional life. Sure they were not that difficult; however, it was easy to doubt the accuracy and degree of completion of the papers. They were not as straight-forward and clear as I had believed they would be. And there was always a large pile of work to do on my desk.

After eight miserable months working with the health insurance company, I decided to return full-time to psychotherapy with my former employer. My boss pitied me after seeing me scratch and claw at the front door, and throwing rocks to try to get his attention. We still joke about this. He was gracious enough to take me back; I felt very good that he had wanted me to return. I felt refreshed and renewed. After the insurance company, I looked forward to seeing my colleagues, doing clinical work, and building up my practice again. I have been happy about this decision ever since.

I had learned that at the insurance company job that there was a vast database collected for each individual, even if the treatment was not covered. And hundreds of people had access to this information. Previously, I spoke about the secretiveness of mental illness. Well, let me tell you, that is only true about individuals who could and maybe should know about your difficulties. It is not true about third party corporations who possess so much personal information about you, data scrutinized to determine the "medical necessity" of your treatment at any particular time. I wish that there did not have to be a third party involved in any person's health care. But, I don't have a better solution other than obtaining parity for mental health coverage.

Chapter 19

OVERRESPONSIBILITY

One night after a long day at work, I called a friend to see if he wanted to go to a bar with someone else and me. Somehow, the topic of Hooters restaurant came up. This topic frequently arises in conversation with us manly men, but on this occasion he expressed disgust. Dread and horror permeated the phone lines because men could wait on tables at Hooters! *What a sacrilege! How could a place called Hooters have men work?* After pointing out this absurdity, I jokingly commented that maybe they would have to change the name to Testes or Packages for the impending hordes of female patrons. As soon as I said the "new" names of Hooters restaurant, I worried that maybe my friend thought that I was gay. *Why else would I say Testes and Packages? Real men don't do that.* My friend's repulsive response to such a revolution in men's "gourmet" eating habits added to my anxiety. It was an anxiety that reminded me when I used to obsess often about my sexuality. The anxiety gradually diminished. Then I called another friend to invite him out for a "guy's night out," but a strange, unfamiliar computer voice asked me to leave a message. I felt uncomfortable about leaving a message because I did not hear his name or voice on the other end. Anybody would have felt uneasy. When I sensed that there was the possibility that I had made a mistake and dialed a wrong number, I started to berate myself and become anxious.

At this point, I felt emotionally dazed and overwrought. Meanwhile, I was uncertain whether I had stepped on the edge of the rug in the living room two minutes before. "Who cares? So what if I had?" I told myself; despite my logical rebuttal to my mental itch, a remnant of emotional pain and angst from the rug incident layered on top of the preexisting anxiety about my sexuality. Telling myself to, "Go with the flow," "Bring on the anxiety," and "Nobody watching me would have known or worried about my shoe possibly teetering on the edge, so I don't need to worry about it," helped me get into a more helpful and less defensive posture about the recent "blunders."

Later that evening, I met my friend at a local watering hole. During our conversation at the bar, the topic of my friend's ex-girlfriend came up (he would say "regurgitated"). Aware of the pain that he had suffered when he had found out that she had been unfaithful, I avoided mentioning her name, but admitted that I was curious if he had heard from her or heard anything about her. He replied that he had received one neutral snippet from a mutual friend. Anyone could see that he continued to be angry with her and that she was a topic that he would talk about as long as he made the rules for the conversation. He went on and on about how he had gotten over her and had found new vitality and energy in his life.

Next, I said something that I had never told my friend. I had thought it for a long time, and had even discussed it with my wife, but never with him, until then. I said something like, "When you first started dating, I never envisioned that the two of you would ever last seven years." Naturally, he wanted to know why. "The two of you are so different. I know opposites attract, but I thought that there were too many differences." As my mouth allowed the sound of the words to come out, I had a vague, pesky feeling that something was not right. I must have offended him in some way. I was afraid that he felt bad about not foreseeing the future of his relationship with her. Underlying my anxiety about what I said to him were the ever-present fears of not having done enough and feeling overresponsible. Maybe I could have forewarned him and saved him from the anguish he had experienced during the three or four years since their breakup.

After saying what I did, my friend inquired why I had not previously informed him about my thoughts regarding his relationship. I did not know. *Oh, no! He thinks that I messed up. He would not ask this question unless he believed that I had screwed up in my duties as a friend.* I told him that he probably would not have paid much attention to my ideas even if I had said something. He was in the relationship too deep and things appeared to be going too well to listen to my relational analysis. He stated that I was likely correct that his behavior would not have changed even if I had asserted my position. His claim to inflexibility did not soothe my discomfort. In fact, I asked him ten minutes later if everything was fine. In addition, I called him two weeks later solely to ascertain the status of our friendship. I feared that he held a grudge against me and did not want to speak to someone so mean and unthoughtful. However, in reality, he reported to me years later, while I was writing this book, that he was already over Jennifer when we talked a few years before. Again, blowing things out of proportion and fearing the worst, in spite of no real evidence to the contrary, emerged as a means to reach the truth. Enormous amounts of anxiety hid the truth, together with a feeling of overresponsibility, and an assumption that an innocent question would be misinterpreted.

The litigiousness of our society has blurred the line that discerns who is responsible for what. Common sense seems to have disappeared, replaced by familiar, ubiquitous warnings about who's fault it is for acting in a certain way. Everyone now knows that McDonald's coffee is very hot (and we did not know this before!). We all live defensively in the hopes of not getting a lawsuit handed to us, sometimes by someone who tries to exploit the system. All of our definitions of responsibility have been challenged and sometimes changed. It is no wonder that anyone, in this era of excessive concern about who is to blame for what, would have difficulty feeling overresponsible. My OCD grew in the fertile ground of uncertainty and doubt of blame. This makes sense because of my conscientious, sensitive, and perfectionistic proclivities.

The scariest incident that I ever experienced with feelings of overresponsibility occurred just a few hours before computers were supposed to go haywire and lead to the end of civilization. The year 2000 (Y2K) rapidly approached.

During the day on New Years Eve, I walked to the local ABC store to pick up some champagne for the upcoming festivities. On my way home, still walking on the strip mall's sidewalk, I noticed that a man twenty yards ahead was sitting down on the sidewalk, his back against a brick wall. Approaching the man, I observed that he appeared motionless with his head facing toward the side. I did not know if he was asleep, unconscious, drunk, or just resting. Others strolled by him with no apparent worry. Nobody stopped to look at or examine him. A man was very close to him talking on the pay phone. *But he's busy chatting. Maybe he doesn't see the man sitting. Maybe nobody does, and I am the only one who does.*

I came within ten yards of the man, but did not learn anything new. I was completely swamped by feelings and thoughts that reflected my ambivalence and vexation. *What should I do? Is the man OK? Is he drunk? That idea makes sense because of how close we are to the ABC store. Worse yet, maybe he's dead.*

I paused for two seconds and then continued for another fifty feet up the sidewalk. Two opposing psychic magnets pulled on the part of my brain that makes decisions. *What do I do? Should I go back and check him and maybe call for an ambulance? The phone is right there? Or should I simply go home?* Unable to mentally resolve the problem and to tolerate the tremendous psychic pain, I returned to the man to have another look. Of course, this checking ritual resulted in more unnecessary anxiety, not less. More because the stakes were so high; I perceived that life and death were in the balance and that it was **incumbent upon me** to choose whether the person would indeed survive. For goodness sake, I doubted if he was alive! Of course, I learned nothing more than I knew before when I looked at the man a second time.

Fortunately, I did not return to him anymore. I figured he was very intoxicated and was sleeping it off. It helped a little to realize that other people did not act as though this was an emergency. I resisted the temptation to look in the obituary section to see if the man had actually died. For two weeks, I experienced varying degrees of anxiety, doubted my (in)action, and prayed for the man.

I recall this incident because I could have let a man die. This is why OCD is as powerful as it is. Catastrophic things do happen (rarely, though, and less frequently if you take reasonable precautions) and life as one knows it could change forever. I could not live the same way feeling extremely guilty. I helped myself by recognizing that my "overresponsibility" OCD was the cause of my excessive anxiety. I also helped myself by continuing to expose myself to the outdoors, stores, people, and the strip mall where I saw the man. During times of excessive anxiety, I was aware that little slices of the world appeared overly dangerous and threatening to me. I was not going to let my hair-trigger nervous system make me behave as though I believed that the world was as dangerous and threatening as I felt. Fortunately, OCD and my feelings about the episode do not cause bad things to happen.

I have also felt overresponsible in my professional role as well as in other areas of my life. In one case, the fear was that maybe by committing an error, the client and the family were not being served as they deserved to be, and as a result they had a more negative attitude towards therapy, therefore rendering it less effective. Perhaps they believed that I was not devoted to the case. *Why shouldn't they think this*? And worst of all, what if the client did not return to therapy with me because of a mistake or oversight, and then decided to never try therapy <u>ever</u> again? The client's pain and suffering that he or she endured for the rest of his or her life would all be my fault!! (notice the "What if" question that unnecessarily raise anxiety.)

This obsession sometimes emerged when I scheduled appointments. I always made my own appointments and kept track of the dates and times of upcoming sessions. I never had a personal secretary at my disposal. (Nor am I asking for one.) Consequently, I was the person who had to take responsibility for any blunders. On rare occasions, I double-booked clients. When this happened, I believed that I committed more scheduling errors than most therapists. In fact, sometimes I convinced myself that I erred more than any other practicing, living therapist. As mentioned before in the book, I tended to engage in all-or-nothing, right vs. wrong dichotomous thinking, a propensity that clearly and unnecessarily increased my anxiety. My elevated anxiety must have confirmed my belief that there was something deficient and inadequate about myself in this one important area. On the contrary, it only signaled that the way I was thinking was distorted and unreasonable, not that I was incompetent and unprofessional. Everybody made mistakes. .

When there was miscommunication between a client and me, I was greatly embarrassed. Having two clients present at the same time for an appointment used to send me into a strong, lasting obsessive state. I <u>was</u> responsible for the mix-up. Being a person who tended to feel overresponsible, this was a very difficult situation for me. I would apologize profusely and typically did not charge him or her for the next session. Most clients and their families realized that everyone made mistakes, even therapists. The majority of my clients took it in stride without getting very upset. I believed that they felt empathy for me in my awkward position. I framed the set of circumstances as an opportunity for the client to practice accepting an imperfect, fallible human being, me. Many of my clients were very hard on themselves for making mistakes and needed to learn how to adapt to unexpected events. Ironically, I had modeled how a person had come to terms with messing up and how to move on afterwards.

During my initial months and years as a therapist, I slowly but steadily changed my perspective of a mistake from being something to be ashamed and guilty about to something from which to learn. I explored and constructed new strategies to make it less likely that the same error occurred again, and if it did, that it would not cause the same heightened level of anxiety.

I realized that I really was not the only therapist who messed up in the stated fashion. I observed other professionals committing errors, too! Once, my former therapist, whose office was in her home, was wearing her pajamas when I knocked on her door. I wondered if perhaps she was trying to make me feel better about my imperfections by intentionally staging this mix-up. She did not purposefully act this way, but it certainly had the same effect. I spoke to other therapists who also disliked the paperwork and administrative parts of their jobs, and who missed or double-booked appointments from time to time. Currently, I give myself permission to make three administrative errors each year. Mistakes happen and I will be ready for them.

Focusing excessively on details and the minutiae of administrative work, even if it was important at times, made it more difficult to concentrate about the genuinely important things that required more attention, the progress of my cases. (I could focus on my cases; it just took a little more energy.) My mind guided me to a task I had more control over. I could not change or control people as I could a pencil and paper. Cases were messy and complicated, filled with ambiguity and uncertainty. In contrast, I could accurately schedule clients and fill out the paperwork almost all of the time. I learned different strategies to assist me to eliminate administrative mistakes. But more importantly, I learned to react to inevitable screw-ups with increased self-tolerance and without self-loathing.

Chapter 20

MAYHEM IN MEXICO

It was our eighth wedding anniversary and we had never been apart on that special date, but on this anniversary I happened to be on a trip with some friends. Lynn and I typically went to a classy restaurant to celebrate, but we wouldn't have the opportunity to do so. I told her that I would call her on the big day. Though separated by thousands of miles, at least we could express our love for one another for a few minutes.

I went with my friends to a restaurant. We had just sat down to rest our legs and to contemplate what to eat when I remembered that I wanted to make a call back to Maryland. A waiter told me that the nearest telephone was outside on the street. They didn't have one inside the building on which to make a long-distance call. So I put my menu back on the table, turned to tell my friends where I was going, and sauntered into the sunlight. I was thinking about what I wanted to say to Lynn. Since I was in the downtown area of Mexico City, it was very busy with people traveling in cars and walking the streets, oblivious to what a gringo was doing there. I walked approximately fifty feet on the sidewalk, crossed the street, and reached the closest pay telephone. I was carefully reading the instructions in English on the phone.

Then, a tall, middle-aged Caucasian man approached me, speaking loudly and gesticulating wildly. Upon reaching me, the man inquired in English about my ability to speak Spanish. I could speak enough to get around and converse some with people. My response pleased him. I wondered why he appeared so upset. He began describing the predicament that had caused his histrionics.

He claimed that his name was Sam and that he was a lawyer who worked at a prestigious financial company in New York City. He said someone had stolen his briefcase, passport, money, and credit cards scarcely fifteen minutes before. He needed to get back to New York the next morning for a very important court date and his airline ticket departed with all his other important personal effects. I felt transported back to work, listening to my clients' struggles.

Because of his apparent sincerity, I listened carefully to his plight. I have always prided myself in successfully interpreting nonverbal behavior and getting a feel for people's motives. He seemed very worried about the circumstances confronting him and angry about his misfortune and the acts of the thieves. I became concerned about him and started to believe that no one else in Mexico City could help him due to the language barrier, the urgency and importance of his call for help, and the difficulty finding someone else who would care enough to help him. In hindsight, my narcissistic needs were met. At work, I had learned the warning signs of this thinking; one begins to feel that because of his or her matchless and trusting relationship with a client, that he or she is the best or the only one that can help a sufferer. My narcissism had diminished with experience, yet it still surfaced to a smaller and more manageable degree, especially when I felt uniquely qualified to help someone. This happened now and then, particularly when a client knew that I was a recovering OCD sufferer. With experience and supervision came less narcissistic thinking. However, I was in the heart of Mexico City in the spring of 2003. I didn't have my supervisor or other colleagues with me there to challenge my unrealistic thinking.

Suddenly, my mind snapped back to my friends. I'd better get back to them or else they would wonder what happened to me. To this day, I hate being the guy who holds people up, someone who causes others to worry. I don't like being the center of attention, either.

But wait, this man is in need. I am a person who likes helping others and this man needed my help, and needed it immediately. *A Good Samaritan doesn't leave anybody behind, particularly someone who asked for help. People don't help each other enough in this world, I don't want to be that way.* Despite not understanding everything that Sam stated regarding telecommunications, wiring money, computers, the U.S. Embassy, and modern technology in general, I strongly believed that he needed **my** help. It certainly sounded like he needed my help. According to him, the U. S. Embassy had not done anything to help, therefore I thought that I needed to do something. If I were in his shoes, I would hope and pray that a kind soul would help me in my time of need. *We're in Mexico for goodness sake! That's a long way from his home in New York City.* I decided that I was going to help Sam, no matter what. My beliefs and value system, core components of my personality, guided me to this conclusion. I wasn't thinking about my friends. I was completely focusing on doing a good deed.

OCD added another layer of factors that contributed to my behavior. I despised feeling that I was not doing enough and that I should have been doing more. My anxiety swelled as I felt very responsible; fear of overresponsibility was my primary obsessional theme that surfaced from time to time. My OCD wanted me to do something to quell the discomfort. Spurred on by my "overresponsibility" anxiety and feeling uncertain about how much time and energy I would need to spend with Sam, I felt marked uneasiness and confusion as we walked through the business center of Mexico City, looking for an "appropriate" bank (according to Sam). As time passed, I became more anxious and apprehensive about walking with Sam. I didn't know where we were or our destination. I began doubting the veracity of Sam's statements.

My friends warned me that Mexico City was rife with predators, ready to exploit unwitting victims at any time. They had traveled a great deal more and had spent time in undeveloped countries where theft was rampant and trust was not an easily earned commodity. In these societies, one must constantly question others' motives. On the other hand, I have lived a cloistered, protected middle-class life and have not been exposed much to the criminal side of human nature. I thought that my friends were well-meaning but overreacting to potential dangers. I never overreact to anything!! Yeah, right. Only when I don't need to.

Paradoxically, I oftentimes perceive that others are overreacting. I have learned that this assumption many times serves the function of reducing my anxiety. The consequences of not listening and incorporating others' concerns about illegal activity in Mexico City (including a woman on the airplane, when I was on my way to Mexico, warning me about potential dangers) were severe and perhaps could have been fatal. Yes, I said fatal. I did not realize it at the time while I was singularly preoccupied with his well-being (and not mine!), that Sam and I were in an isolated area at one point, removed from people. Who knows what he had planned for me if I had not provided him with enough money to buy a plane ticket? (I learned later that an accomplice was nearby, someone who quickly picked him up in a car after the entire encounter ended.) After he left me, I realized that I was fortunate to have given him a large amount of money. Ironically, this might have saved my life or kept me from harm.

Back at the restaurant, I found out later that my friends were very worried about me since I was nowhere to be found. People were very frightened for my well-being. They knew that I was not at the closest outdoor telephone or anywhere within a one- block radius of the restaurant. My friend's mother cried and the police were called to determine what had transpired. The largest newspaper in Mexico City carried a small story about me in the next day's edition!

Learning about the impact that my behavior had on others later that day, I hated my intrusive thoughts and images of my friends crying, pacing, and worrying about me. I obsessed about how my actions had caused others to feel. I was largely responsible for how they felt, but I was (and continued later) feeling overresponsible, worrying that I had caused irreparable emotional trauma to my friends. It was actually very emotionally traumatic for everyone; my friends were not overreacting. I had used very poor judgment and scared them half-to-death (maybe this explains the origin of this expression). I was so preoccupied and single-minded in purpose to provide aid to the man that I had discounted and denied the reaction that my friends were likely to have. I told myself, "They know I'm fine. They just figure that I am still talking to my wife. Since it is our anniversary, they know it will be a long conversation. I'll be right back. They are busy eating anyway." Clearly, I was not thinking reasonably.

Two hours had passed with Sam! I was safe but lost in Mexico City, emotionally and physically disoriented and consumed with self-doubt. I seriously doubted the intelligence of what I had just done, especially after seeing the man quickly get into a car after we had departed ways. The two hours flew by rapidly due to my "overresponsibility" OCD with helping the man, and my vacation rule of never wearing a watch. I went extremely out of my way to help Sam, doing things that I now revisit and shake my head at. To make the story short (and minimize the damage to my ego), my friends and I met up later back at our hotel. I felt horrible because people truly believed that something terribly wrong had happened to me. My friend's concern, irritation, and vexation stared me directly in the face. And all I had wanted to do was to help somebody.

My friends and I went to another person's house. There, everyone discussed my odyssey and wanted to know what happened and why I had not returned to the restaurant to tell them what I was doing. There was no good, rational reason why I did not tell my friends. It did not feel comfortable and self-respecting to say anything at the house but it was impossible to remain silent. I tried to explain the circumstances surrounding my actions, attempting to make sense of the whole crazy mess. Opening my mouth only served to clarify what I knew deep down; I had really made a huge mistake, and there was no way to fix it or redo it. I obsessed about making small mistakes, so during this entire episode my anxiety had reached one of the highest points ever. I was holding out hope that the man was going to pay me back for purchasing his airplane ticket, but in my heart I knew that Sam had stolen money from me that I would never see again. He had given me his name, address, phone number, and other "relevant" information. The longer that I spoke to my friends, the more I was convinced that Sam had taken advantage of me.

We drove eight hours that night to Guadalajara. I displaced anger directed towards the unscrupulous man and myself and yelled at my friend. I hardly ever yell at anybody. He was insightful enough to know that I was angry because I was aware of my mistakes. His interpretation was accurate, but it increased my anger and anxiety. Anxiety because I never desired my faults and shortcomings to surface, especially in such a public manner. I wanted to bury myself under the seat, never to reappear again. Better yet, I wanted to be back home doing anything other than sitting in the van. The van held me captive and forced me to talk and hear what others were saying. I spoke more defensively than ever and was short with my friends. It was eight hours of recounting the sequence of events and engaging in mental activity with the goal to reason with myself and conclude that Sam would indeed return the funds. (I played a game called Mental Sisyphus.) I engaged in much self-loathing. It was the longest trip known to mankind. I was too anxious and angry to go to sleep or to drive. I was awake the entire trip, staring out the window and looking at the foreboding sky, wishing that this was not an omen of more ignominious incidents on the dark horizon. The sky looked as I felt.

I not only made a huge error in judgment and emptied my wallet of hundreds of dollars, but my friends discovered the truth about me. Ripping my mask off, this incident, unlike any other, had shown others my weaknesses. I could and did make big mistakes; I had messed up in a major way. Trying previously not to make mistakes from time to time, I believe I became more human to them that day. My vulnerabilities had been exposed, and I was feeling and acting uncharacteristically. Taking anything positive away from what had occurred, I believed that I became more human to my friends.

Everything turned out all right. I even got to talk to my panic-stricken wife later that night. I was fine (at least physically) and money could always be replaced. I am a little wiser now. Most importantly, I realize that not heeding the warnings of others can be dangerous, and that I must be more aware of my vulnerabilities and personal proclivities. The man had exploited my firm belief that helping others should be everyone's priority, no matter under what circumstances. However, awareness alone is not sufficient; I need to behave differently to reinforce this lesson. Recognition that OCD can shift and even tip the balance from acting wisely to behaving imprudently and recklessly is another hard lesson learned. When OCD is linked with a personality "blind spot," the combination can lead to undesired outcomes. Over time, I have significantly improved with this mixture. Sam got me this time. I vow that no one will catch me in a similar emotionally-compromised position again. And by the way, don't ask me for change!

Chapter 21

REVIEW AND WORDS OF WISDOM

My OCD has changed dramatically over the years. Writing this book has permitted me to discover precisely how much. Thankfully, there have been major improvements. My symptomatology has substantially decreased and my ability to cope with OCD is much greater. When OCD arrived on the scene in Dr. Judith Rapoport's The Boy Who Couldn't Stop Washing, I was counting numbers in my head. Today, the only numbers in my consciousness appear when I reconcile my checkbook and when I'm at the store calculating which brand of detergent is the least expensive. Numbers come to me only when they are welcome and useful. Likewise, I used to get extremely anxious when I masturbated as a teenager, even obsessing that someone up on the neighbor's roof would certainly discover my abominable behavior. Now, my wife and I enjoy a healthy, satisfying sex like. For goodness sake, the secret's out with two children! There's no doubt that I have enjoyed intimacy with my wife at least twice. Furthermore, I don't obsess and get compulsive about whether I've disposed of the evidence "well enough." I see self-stimulation for what it is, not a sin or self-abuse and not something to be ashamed of or guilty about, but something to enjoy.

In my teenage years and early twenties, I was so concerned about what others thought of me as if they, and not I, defined my worth. I now realize that I'm a rather nice, reserved, thoughtful, and analytic guy who generally feels good about himself. If one of my friends would rather do something else than have me come over and hang out, I don't take it personally. Another vital skill I learned was to let people know if they've said something hurtful. Being assertive, I can tease the teaser, making fun of an inconsiderate person's powerlessness to push my buttons. I constantly remind myself, "Don't take yourself so seriously. Loosen up." In earlier times, my lack of a response generally contributed to elevated levels of anxiety and a sense that my "bad" emotions led to passive behavior. Speaking up and standing up for myself was difficult; however, my long-term anxiety levels diminished and my self-confidence soared.

The most painful and distressing obsession was my fear of being or acting in a homosexual manner. I couldn't watch television or see a guy without wondering about my sexuality. Currently, I rarely experience thoughts about the possibility of being or becoming homosexual. In fact, recognition of a man's good looks does not send me over the obsessional edge as it once did. Certainly, living with my wife for twelve years has significantly reduced these doubts.

I have learned a great deal about how to cope with long-term obsessions. Many of these strategies are useful at any time with OCD. As stated earlier, starting at 10:40 A.M. on September 15, 1982, I began having long-term or "distant" obsessions. A very pertinent question is, "How do I get from OCDing to not OCDing about a certain theme that originated years ago. Acceptance of incoming thoughts and anxiety, examining them as if I were a news reporter, is very helpful. Looking at my thoughts rather than getting caught up in my thoughts is very important. I make a habit of not overreacting to the anxiety; my emotions don't get the best of me. For example, sometimes, I obsess about and engage in mental rituals about old themes that have not presented themselves for months or even years. For some strange, unknown reason, I may wonder if I looked at a guy in the wrong way. Perhaps he would misinterpret my actions. (Thankfully, this ridiculous obsession emerges rarely now.) I remind myself that my OCD sometimes goes back in time when I am under more stress. I don't engage in self-pity or get depressed about the situation. I simply watch what is transpiring with my mind's eye and don't make any judgments about myself. I tell myself that this is OCD and not to give it any more relevance and meaning. This is a form of exposure since I am paying attention to the fear, but in addition, I am paying attention to all my sensory input and what feelings and thoughts I have. I am being mindful of what is transpiring in that exact moment.

Second, I need to revisit the source of my anxiety many times. I need to combat the OCD on my terms and not take for granted that a specific symptom has been eliminated even if OCD about the distant past has not surfaced for a few days. Many sufferers can usually perform the necessary exposure exercises during everyday activities without necessarily using a special, discrete block of time to perform exposures. E/RP is the most powerful tool that we have in our tool belt. It will not help much to raise my anxiety sporadically, too briefly, or in a haphazard, disjointed, abrupt fashion; or to react to the OCD instead of attacking it head-on.

Third, I have found that it helps to see the old, stale obsessional theme from a new, fresh perspective. A new way of thinking may help to infuse some humor and may inspire a different view of the world and of the events that led to the long-term obsession. Sufferers often get stuck in irrational, unreasonable thought patterns. For me, an overresponsible obsessive-compulsive, the statement "Sometimes doing nothing is doing something" has been very useful. Of course, sometimes doing nothing is still doing nothing. Sometimes a cigar is just a cigar.

Finally, the passing of time helps the pain to dwindle. I try to remember that there will not be a smooth, gradual amelioration of symptoms over time. Sometimes you go back a step to advance two. Positive involvement in life distracts the mind and pushes out longstanding obsessions. Time does heal, but it is not a good plastic surgeon. That is why it is so important to receive treatment early after the onset of OCD. Receiving treatment provides the best chance of achieving the most successful outcome.

The course of OCD is somewhat predictable in the sense that symptoms generally increase in frequency, intensity, and duration as a consequence of psychosocial stressors. The days leading up to my graduations and wedding were days of very high anxiety. It is important to note that my anxiety does not always increase when it "should." There are occasions when others around me are panicking and I wonder why they are reacting in this fashion. I reframe my problems as opportunities. On account of frequently feeling anxious, I am more prepared to cope with difficult times in life. There are times when anxiety surfaces seemingly from out of nowhere. The most frustrating thing for a sufferer is to experience problems even if life is not particularly stressful or overwhelming. The absolute worst time for a symptom to appear is while on vacation.

My symptoms reflect my current developmental stage and life roles. For example, during puberty I obsessed about feeling guilty about masturbating. As a teenager, discovering my sexuality and my body and feeling new, awkward, insecure, and anxious, I obsessed about this subject. Of course, I'm not going to obsess about this theme now when I am a middle-aged adult. It doesn't possess the emotional power that it did twenty or thirty years ago when sex was a novel thing. Similarly, I now obsess about uncertainties and emotionally-charged themes in my current position in life. What do you know? I'm now obsessing about whether or not I am performing as well as I should at my job or as a parent. What an amazing coincidence! Being a breadwinner and a father are the two "job" that I have now. Who would have thought that I obsess about my competency and "doing my best" in the two roles I now have? By the way, what does "doing my best" mean? It is a very vague concept that not everyone understands in the same way.

In regards to psychotropics, I have tried numerous medication regimens over the years. Finally, I found the one that worked best for me and I have stuck with it for seven years. Prozac works the best. It is monumentally frustrating to try medication after medication, serving as an involuntary guinea pig. I participated in the early research on Anafranil (Chlorimipramine) in 1982 at the National Institutes of Mental Health. The drug had not yet even been approved for use in the United States at that point. My mother called England at 5 A.M. in order to purchase the medicine. I have taken about every drug known to mankind that could even theoretically decrease OCD symptoms. For example, one doctor suggested that perhaps Depakote, a drug sometimes used for bipolar disorder, might benefit me.

In addition, I recognized this as a medication that I had administered for seizure management to a resident at the group home where I worked. But again, I went along with the doctor. However, as seen in my story, I finally reached a point where I was not willing to try any new medication for any reason. I had become more depressed on one medicine and could barely function on another because I was so sedated. Despite the adverse effects, it is important to keep doing whatever it takes to get the proper help. Eventually you will find the medication that is right for you, as I did.

Presently, I continue to have some mild struggles with doubts and obsessions about my competency at work. I am improving quickly, though, feeling more confident about my ability to assist people as I gain more experience. I have learned emotionally that despite my OCD fears, I really am a good therapist! I have not allowed my OCD to push me around and dictate the parameters of my life. I have remained at my job, exposing myself to much anxiety. (It is exposure because all the evidence suggests that I am adequate and competent at work.) That exposure is paying off, for it is now much easier brushing aside feelings of inferiority and overresponsibility. Sure I make mistakes, and it's OK to make some mistakes because we learn from them. Therapists are human, too. Most significantly, I know that I have faced my fear of being inadequate and overresponsible and have come through it again. I am still a good, worthwhile person even if I do make some mistakes. Come to think of it, making mistakes is a prerequisite to being a fully alive and mature person. It's amazing that people get through it somehow. Stubbornness and persistence serve me well.

If I can manage my OCD, then I know others can, too. I see it every day. The bad times will pass. If there is the presence of secondary depression, the suicidal and hopeless times always pass and we become more productive and hopeful. It many take longer than you want, but it will happen. I haven't been suicidal for more than fifteen years. The teenage years were the toughest for me, as they are for many others. OCD is the cross that I bear, every single day of my life. It's a cross that is very heavy for me on occasion but very light for the majority of the time. Many worse things can befall a person, though it doesn't seem that way while overburdened with obsessions.

Believe me, if anyone knows how difficult OCD is to manage, it is I. Individuals without OCD who have academic and clinical knowledge do not know exactly what you are experiencing. They can't, and they don't have to. You can still be helped if you are willing. Sure, everyone is sometimes somewhat obsessive and compulsive. As any OCD sufferer knows, when you are in the throes of a very intrusive and distressing bout with OCD, it is not an experience that most have had or can understand. OCD has humbled me. It is an enemy with which I have been forced to make my peace. In order to conquer an enemy, we much learn to respect it, yet not allow ourselves to be ruled by it. Disarm your foe with acceptance.

Every day, I decide that I'm going to have a good day in spite of my OCD.

PART III:
IMPACT OF OCD ON OTHERS

Chapter 22

MY PARENTS' VIEWS

The following four chapters in Part III: Impact of OCD on Others discuss OCD in the context of a relationship. On the contrary, in Parts I and II, I narrate and describe my own experiences which are frequently independent of a specific bond. My parents speak first; this part contains some of my important historical data. Then, my wife writes about the impact of OCD on our marriage. Next, I talk about how others, including some of my clients, respond to learning about my diagnosis. Finally, I write about how I think that OCD manifests itself in my marriage.

John was born January 19, 1967 and adopted by us on January 24, 1967 through the Mercer County Social Services of Mercer County, Pennsylvania. My wife and I were excited and thrilled to get this delightful red haired boy. He was the joy of our life and adjusted very quickly. He slept through the night in approximately two weeks and at about that same time, began to take some solid food. Other than this very early development of a night sleep pattern and the willingness to take solid food at an early age, all developmental patterns were normal. As he grew older, he did develop a lot of ear infections that led to tubes being placed in his ears on two occasions. He finally had his tonsils and adenoids removed and that seemed to alleviate the problem.

Sometime in 1980, at about the age of 13, John mentioned to his mother that numbers kept going through his head and he couldn't make it stop happening. We had no knowledge or inclination that this was symptomatic of a major problem, and, in fact, found it difficult to believe. We thought it was simply an indication of an overactive childhood imagination. We did nothing about his complaint and he did not mention it again for over a year. During that time, however, we began to notice changes in his behavior. He had to bathe every day, and if something caused him to miss a day, he became extremely distressed. He spent an inordinate amount of time in the bathroom, almost to the point of monopolizing it. It became a standing family joke. His walk and actions became very slow and deliberate. We thought of these changes as unusual, perhaps even idiosyncratic, and even kidded John about them. Again, we had no reason to believe these behaviors were symptomatic of a major problem. While always somewhat quiet and introverted, John became even more withdrawn.

However, a year after his first symptoms appeared, John again came to his mother, in tears, and said he believed he was going crazy; he needed to see a psychiatrist. He didn't want his mother to say anything about this to anyone, including me, his father. His mother first took him to the family pediatrician who recommended a local psychiatrist whom he believed might be able to help. Upon this recommendation, John's mother convinced him that I needed to know what was going on and John reluctantly agreed. After several visits to the psychiatrist, John was diagnosed with OCD. Following additional discussions with John, we finally convinced him that his brother and sister also needed to know what was going on, as they were quite aware of his seemingly strange behavior and needed to have some idea of what was happening. Again, John reluctantly agreed, but made it clear that no one else was to know, not even his grandparents. The finding of OCD did little for us other than place a name on John's condition. We had a thousand questions. What had caused it? Why did it happen to John? What was the short-term and long-term prognosis? How would it affect John's ability to become a functional adult? Could it be cured? The doctor was able to provide few answers to our questions. Not much was known about OCD at that time, and in fact, little authoritative information was available on the subject. As parents, this was both frustrating and painful. We finally understood, at least to some degree, the pain John was going through and that he was being affected both mentally and physically. We began to understand how seriously depressed John was and how the condition affected his ability to cope with normal day-to-day activities. We hurt to see him hurting. In addition, we felt a lot of guilt in those early days.

Was it somehow our fault that the condition had developed? Why had we ignored it earlier? Why couldn't we have seen that there was a major problem and gotten help for him much earlier than we did? We literally sat down and tried to remember every incident in John's childhood in an attempt to find some answer, some contributing factor. In retrospect, we marvel that John was able to somehow continue attending school, deliver the newspapers early every morning, and do excellent work in each. As mentioned previously, John's early childhood did not seem to indicate anything unusual. If anything, as a child John was better than we were led to believe was possible for a child. He adapted to schedules quickly and easily; he was very cooperative and was rarely disruptive; he did not go through the "terrible two's," in fact, he was a model child in terms of deportment. It was obvious that he wanted to please and tried very hard to do those things that he felt would make us happy with him.

He was also a bright, intelligent child. He began his formal schooling in kindergarten. After approximately two weeks, his teacher called to say that she was recommending he be placed into first grade, as kindergarten was a waste of time for him. We agreed to this, and it was in the first grade that a rare incident of disobedience occurred. The school was having a bake sale. John's mother baked a cake for it and asked John to take it in to school that morning. For whatever reason, he did not want to carry it to school, so shortly after leaving home, he hid it in the bushes. Several weeks later, his mother was out for a walk, happened to look into the bushes, and saw the cake. We sent him in with a donation of money for the school and made him tell the teacher what had happened. To this day we talk about it, and have a good laugh over this with John.

In general, John performed very well academically, though he did not fare so well in the social arena. He had only a couple of really close friends, and tended to get along better with adults than with his peers. As we reflect back on it, under pressure the OCD had a particular effect on John.

John began playing soccer at an early age, for teams at the local Youth Center. He became an excellent soccer player and eventually began playing on a select team. It was at this time that the OCD started to become particularly bad. It did not affect him so much as a club player because he felt no particular pressure to excel. On the select team though, given his skills, his coach expected much. As he felt more and more pressure to perform at a consistently high level, it became more and more difficult for him to do so. As a result of the OCD, when placed in a particularly pressurized situation, he would simply freeze on the field. This behavior would result in his getting yelled at by both his coach and his fellow players, which created even more pressure. Finally, he simply couldn't take it any longer and quit playing.

In addition, as symptoms of OCD began to become more prevalent, John tended to become more withdrawn socially. Although somehow he continued to do very well academically, John did not begin to catch up socially until college. He eventually joined a fraternity and was able to get away from home and live in the fraternity house for a period of six months. While continuing to battle symptoms of OCD, John was able to successfully major in Psychology and graduated with about a B+ average. During that time, he became the facilitator of a local OCD support group. Given his personal experience with OCD, his work with the National Institutes of Mental Health (NIMH), and his work with individuals in the support group, he became very interested in having a career in which he would be able to help others experiencing problems of that nature. This was a major influence on his decision to major in Psychology as an undergraduate. After graduating from George Washington University, he continued his education, earning a Masters of Social Work (MSW) from Virginia Commonwealth University, and is now working as a CBT therapist. We are very proud of his accomplishments.

Unfortunately, all our recollections and soul-searching provided little to help us come to any resolution of our concerns. Certainly, as we looked back, we could see many incidents that provided an indication that all was not well. Yet, we could find nothing that would point to why the problem had developed. While we could not have any idea of what John was going through (one needs to experience it to understand it) we could understand why he was so secretive about it. He felt he was the only person in the world to experience such problems, and he felt utterly isolated and alone. We had that same feeling. We had to suffer in silence, as John would not allow us to share our grief and concerns with our best friends. We didn't know of anyone else that had such a condition.

Then the psychiatrist mentioned that NIMH was beginning studies on OCD and would be testing a new medication that they thought might be effective. The program accepted him. For us, the program was both a God-send and a major disappointment. A disappointment, because we wanted so badly for John to be "cured." We looked for the medication to provide a miracle solution. Of course, it did not. We were scared half to death when told by personnel at NIMH that John was severely depressed and suicidal, and we still remember the suicide watches that were the result of that information. But, in other ways, we may not have been able to survive mentally without it.

The strain of the situation had been particularly bad on John's mother. She simply could not stop feeling that somehow she was to blame for his condition. Consequently, she went into a deep depression, lost weight, and for over a year also received counseling and took antidepressants. Up to that time, she had been a stay-at-home mom, but now she could not stand to be at home alone during the day. It gave her too much time to think, and all she could think about was the suffering that she knew John was going through. Consequently, to keep both mind and body occupied, and secondarily to provide insurance that would have mental health benefits, which would be required for a number of years, she took a job outside the home. She continued to work at that job until her retirement.

The NIMH program also included a support group for the parents. Finally, we could share our worries, our concerns, and our questions with experts and with others feeling the same concerns. Because of those seminal studies, OCD began to be less secretive, more was learned about it, and a variety of medications and CBT regimens were developed which had benefits for some individuals. Newspaper articles, pamphlets, journal articles, and books were published. Most of all, individuals with OCD and those that love and care about them found that they were not alone. We learned that many others suffer some manifestation of the disorder.

Along with John's involvement with the OCD self-help group, came many calls funneled through our house giving us the opportunity to talk with other individuals who had OCD, or with their parents. We learned more about the condition, and as usual, with knowledge comes, if not understanding, at least a realization that neither John nor we probably could have done anything to prevent the condition from occurring. We were able to find some personal peace with ourselves. In addition, we gained a better understanding of what

John was coping with just in trying to deal with what most of us would consider normal, everyday activities. It made us even more amazed at what he has been able to accomplish, and provides some evidence that, at least in particular instances, and with help, an individual with OCD can be a productive and accomplished individual, even though they may go through a kind of personal hell in trying to do it.

Since the time we first learned of John's condition, John and we have come a long way. John is engaged in what would seem to be a very successful career, doing what he wants to do, which is to help others. He is married to a wonderful young woman, and they are parents of two marvelous children. Most importantly, and the focus of this book, is that no one needs to go through the years of misery, depression, and feeling of isolation that John and we did. Help is available. All one needs to do is reach out for it.

Chapter 23

MY WIFE'S VIEWS

John and I met at work. I was pleasantly surprised when he called and asked me to lunch. Our first date was at a restaurant called Bennigan's; I felt that we clicked from the start. We laughed a lot on that date and I loved his sense of humor. One thing he said really stuck in my mind. We were on the topic of relationships, and he mentioned how so many people don't persist long enough or stick through things together these days. I thought that to be very true. We continued to date, and I found myself liking him more and more.

He used good judgment in determining the right time to tell me about his OCD. We were just getting close to each other, but weren't so far into the relationship that I felt like he was hiding something. Had he told me on our first date, I honestly think I would have been scared off. I remember very clearly the night that he told me. He was open and honest with me.

He told me that he'd had OCD since he was a teenager; he described what OCD was. He said that since he had obsessions and not overt compulsions, I probably wouldn't notice a whole lot. I felt a tremendous amount of compassion for him, as well as feeling somewhat scared by this information. I had heard of OCD, and always associated it with handwashing or compulsive cleaning. I must admit that I wondered what I was getting myself into. I decided to find out more about OCD and did some reading, as well as asking John more about his particular symptoms. I found myself constantly looking for behaviors. At first I didn't notice much, mostly because he had obsessions/compulsions that couldn't be seen.

I was falling in love with John. I decided at that point that the OCD didn't seem to affect the relationship much, and I wanted to continue to see him. As we got closer, I began to notice that when he obsessed he was more distant and preoccupied. He also moved slower at doing things when his anxiety was high. These things were subtle, but more noticeable the better I got to know him. I went through many phases where I would get scared, wonder if I was fooling myself, and think that OCD might profoundly affect a relationship with him. I found myself really wanting to understand, but having a difficult time with it.

At that time, he was leading an OCD support group. There was a Family and Friends group that met at the same time. I thought about going to it, but felt that I wouldn't be able to talk openly with them knowing him as the leader of the other group. I also felt that I didn't know where "girlfriend" fit in the group. Looking back, this seems ridiculous, but at the time it seemed to make sense. I went through a phase of feeling as if I might cause him to obsess by something I would say or do. John was always good about not letting me enable him to ritualize. He did not ask reassuring questions. I definitely did not want to answer any OCD questions.

I can see how easily people can fall into the role of "enabler." You love someone and hate to see him or her in pain. You know that if it's something you're doing that's raising their anxiety, then you can change it and they'll feel better. With OCD though, this is the worst thing you can do, because it will actually worsen things in the long run. I began thinking a lot about enabling behaviors and tried to be very conscious not to do them.

The next phase I experienced coming to terms with John's OCD was one of feeling that OCD wasn't real, or that it was an excuse. He would tell me he "wasn't feeling well" (meaning he was obsessing), and that's why he was more "distant" and preoccupied. I noticed many more "distant" times the closer we got. I began to think that the distance I felt reflected a problem between us. I would often think *"He must not be happy with something in the relationship."* *"Maybe he doesn't really love me"*, or *"I am somehow not who he really wants."*

Reflecting on it, I think that I went through a classic stage of denial. It was easier for me to believe it was something that I had done instead of the reality of John's OCD that caused any tension in our relationship. I guessed if it were something I had done, I could change it, but I could not change OCD. This stage, though it got progressively better, carried over into our married life, and occasionally still arises. We've worked extensively on our communication. This is such a vital thing in any relationship, but it is especially so in our case.

We dated for a long period of time. We were young when we met, 21 and 22, and I was still in school. Before he asked me to marry him, I remember both of us really questioning the relationship. I started feeling that he was asking too many questions. I began to wonder if he really felt that it was right or not. He told me that OCD was playing a part in it. I really battled with that within myself, because I felt that if you had to question the relationship that much, then maybe it was not meant to be. We went to see his therapist together, and one thing that came out was that my weight bothered him. That really hurt, because I've always been very sensitive about my weight. At that time I was slightly overweight, but not by much. It <u>was</u> bothering me, and I felt that I wanted to lose some weight. I began to feel, though, that if he couldn't love me for who I was, then I didn't want to be with him.

In pre-marital therapy, we both learned that John was working through his feelings about marriage and looking for any of my possible flaws. His perfectionism, elevated anxiety levels, and my own insecurities about my weight were contributing to the conflict. This was a difficult time; I wondered if I was a fool to believe that John's perfectionism and high anxiety were affecting the situation, or if other non-clinical factors impinged upon our relationship. I never wanted to feel that I was just settled on, and not what he really wanted in a wife. I felt I deserved better than that. I began to realize that it was very difficult to distinguish between normal everyday feelings and OCD. It really confused me. Was there a real and understandable reason for his doubt, or was he hiding behind the cloak of OCD and perfectionism?

I felt terribly distant from him when he was obsessing, but at other times, I felt very close. I was in love with him and felt he had become one of my very best friends. I remember writing in my diary about all my intense feelings, and working out whether to continue in the relationship. We actually spent a week apart without any contact to see how we felt. I hated not talking to him and missed him a lot. I realized how much I really loved and wanted him in my life. The respite was a big turning point for me. I realized that I had a choice. I was in no way stuck in the relationship.

I chose to be with him and to accept that OCD would always be there. OCD certainly did not define John, and I loved who he was in spite of his OCD. I knew that I wanted to stick by him, through the good times and the bad. I felt that I could learn to deal with those times in which I felt distant from him. It took him a little while after this to propose. I wondered why it took him so long. *Was there something wrong with our relationship?*

We had a wonderful wedding and an even better honeymoon. I knew that I had done the right thing. Our first year was somewhat difficult because we were still working on some of the premarital issues. After that first year, I think we emerged with a much deeper understanding and love for each other.

Bringing children into our relationship was a big step. We planned on having both our daughter Elizabeth, and our son Christopher. When we started trying to conceive, I could sense John's anxiety. It was interesting because his OCD definitely worsened around this big life event. Those types of situations are still hard for me, because I wonder how much of his heightened anxiety is caused by OCD, and how much is normal anxiety about a given life event. I worried how it would be with a baby, if the added stress and responsibilities would "throw him over the edge."

I got pregnant right away. We were both so excited. He began to have some anxieties about sex and hurting the baby. It's interesting looking back on that time because I think we weren't communicating as clearly. I was worried about him not liking the weight that I had gained, but he was genuinely worried about hurting the baby. I couldn't see the OCD part of it at that time. I thought for sure that he just wasn't telling me to spare my feelings. We did finally work it through, and we both eventually felt better about it. I can definitely see the pattern now. It's some form of denial mixed with my own insecurities that make it tough for me. If it's me bringing about the problem, that's something tangible; I can comprehend this situation and do something about it. But if it's the OCD, it's intangible and nothing I can fix or change. I am better able to acknowledge and understand my true feelings about a situation. As time passes, it takes a lot of communication about what each of us is really feeling to know how to improve our behavior toward each other.

While I was pregnant, John went through a phase when his OCD was bad and he was wondering about changing jobs. His OCD centered on his work at that time. This really scared me, mostly because being pregnant I wanted security, as most women would. I was afraid that he wouldn't be able to work because of his OCD. I've found that he goes through these phases every once in awhile; I realize now that he wouldn't quit his job without having another one in line. If he did get to the point where he couldn't work, it certainly wouldn't be ideal, but we would get the best help available for him and we would manage. One of the things that amazes me about John is that even though there are a lot of rough times, he always manages to get back on his feet again. He never gives up in situations when I think many other people would. He's a special person in that sense.

Becoming parents has been an amazing and wonderful challenge. Our children, Elizabeth and Christopher, are such blessings in our lives. Currently, John is working full- time and I am working part-time. We both value being present and involved with our children. When he's working I'm home with the kids, and when I'm working he's home with them. It's such a juggling act! We both have more responsibilities and less down time. I used to be able to give more support to John during his tough times, but now there are three people to focus on, so my attention is divided between them.

I think that John's OCD affects me as a parent especially when I feel tired and stressed (and what parent doesn't from time to time!). At those times, I feel like I need more support and help with the kids. It used to be hard for me to ask for what I needed, but I am much better at it now. Once again, the issue of communication is vital. I was always scared that asking for help, especially when he was in his state of "not feeling well" (high anxiety) would "throw him over the edge." I've come to realize that not requesting help, because of his elevated anxiety, is actually enabling John's OCD to win. When I don't ask for what I need, I get overwhelmed and cannot be of real use to anyone. Importantly, I have found that he is not that fragile, and that he is willing to pitch in if I point out to him what the needs are. **He can't read my mind!** (darn!) He may not always feel like doing something when his OCD is flaring up (e.g. a chore at home, running an errand, etc.), but it doesn't break him, and he will help with prompting. We are working on defining our roles and responsibilities, which certainly helps decrease tension between us. In any relationship, and especially with young children, it's vital to help and support one another. A healthy marriage should be a partnership, with both people doing their share and contributing to the relationship or it cannot work.

As I mentioned before, communication has turned out to be a key issue. We found that if he told me more about his obsessions and what he experienced internally, I felt more connected, and was better able to give him the space he needed. I used to reach out to him more physically, through touch, etc. This was the last thing he wanted when he was obsessing; I felt that he further distanced himself from me. I didn't know any other way to connect with him though, because he wasn't emotionally available to me. There's a fine line between being an enabler and being a concerned and supportive wife. It's very helpful knowing what's happening inside of him, though it's important to find the balance of talking enough about it while not making it all of the conversation and focus. It's a line that can be walked (carefully), and it makes a world of difference. I have to say I've developed a deep admiration for John. Knowing more of what goes on inside of him, what he battles with in his mind, and seeing him still able to carry on a fairly normal life amazes me. I have the utmost respect for him. I love him very deeply.

Presently, I find that the emotional distance that OCD creates during his times of high anxiety is harder to deal with. It feels very lonely at times. We used to have more opportunities to reconnect with each other because we had more time, whereas now we don't. We are trying to have a date night once a week to at least try to create that opportunity. That is helpful. We have to make much more of an effort to stay connected. It certainly is worth it! I've found that what *I* can do is: take care of myself; stay healthy; not be an enabler; express my feelings and needs; keep open communication; stay centered and spiritual; and pursue my own interests and hobbies. Then I am able to be more supportive and have much more to give everyone. I wouldn't change life with children for the world. I think both of our lives are richer because of these little angels we've been blessed with. We just have to never give up on each other and keep our connection strong.

Being in a relationship with someone who has OCD has its difficult times, but with work, one realizes that OCD is only one facet of a person, not all of who that person is. It also makes all the difference when the person experiencing it has the will to fight the ongoing battle OCD brings, and attempts to optimize their mental health. Without that aspect, I don't think a relationship would have much of a chance of working. I can never imagine being married to anyone else but John; I'm happy right where I am. I love the expression that the grass is not always greener on the other side, but where you water it. I feel my love for John grow more all the time through our experiences together. We have to remember to keep the grass watered though! Another spin on that as a spouse is for me to remember to let everyone take responsibility for watering their part of the grass, and the times I have to step in and help water, I have to remember to take the time to refill my watering can.

Before we got married, I remember him telling me that he sometimes wondered if I knew what I was getting myself into with him having OCD. I think at that point I had a fairly good idea, though one can never truly know until they've experienced different life circumstances together. I don't feel that I've had any major surprises however. I admit many times I wish it would just go away. I'm sure John does, too. I especially wish this when we go on vacation or go to visit my family and his OCD is bothering him. He tends to keep to himself and sleep more. Vacation and family times are when I most want to have fun with him. Not that he doesn't interact or have fun at all; it's much less than usual though. I find myself feeling somewhat guilty for wishing he didn't have OCD, which I assume is normal. I think it's important to keep in mind that he can't just "will" it away. That's hard to remember sometimes because it's not something you can see, like a broken leg. I do think though that it is important to support healthy behaviors, and not just accept isolation and withdrawal in the rough times.

I worry a lot about not completely understanding John's OCD. I wonder if I'm being supportive enough, or if I'm enabling the OCD to get stronger. I've tried to educate myself about it, and believe I have a pretty good idea of what he must experience. I know I can never completely understand it because I don't have it. I can see sometimes how an obsession presents itself -- it makes some sort of sense. It may be something that I might worry about for a little while, then my mind works it out so that I feel okay and take the appropriate actions to make things right. For John, it seems the mind can't make things okay, it has to hold onto them and worry about them. John has described OCD to me as a "mosquito bite" of the brain. It keeps itching and the more you scratch it, the worse it gets.

In addition to navigating how to live with someone diagnosed with OCD, I am also curious why he has been very hesitant to tell people about OCD. I've always felt that I have to keep "hush-hush" about it. Most of my family and friends don't know about it. When I ask about telling them, he usually says that they really don't need to know; it's not something that affects them. In some instances I agree; however, there have been times that I think it would have been beneficial to tell family and friends. These cases occur when the people I know have loved ones with OCD or similar problems, and sometimes when visiting family. If his OCD is flaring up at the time of a visit, he becomes quieter and more isolated. Some people have wondered then if something is wrong with John, or if they've done something bothersome. I usually say that he's exhausted from work or that it's been a tough week. I feel as if I'm carrying around a big secret or telling a lie. I do agree that not everyone needs to know something like that, but it would be helpful to have family and close friends be able to lend support through the difficult times. In these situations I feel very isolated.

Recently, he has been less hesitant to divulge personal information. This is a good development for both of us. I think that many people can be helped in their own circumstances if they know of someone else that has OCD, who is working on living a functional, full, and meaningful life with it. **This is why I think this book will be so helpful, not only for John and myself, but for many others, too.**

Chapter 24

OCD IN MY RELATIONSHIP WITH LYNN

Despite all evidence that indicated that I was making the best move at the time, I obsessed about the decision whether to marry Lynn. Almost everyone obsesses about whether or not the person he or she is supposed to marry is the "right" person, whatever that means. This obsession is typically and usually adaptive to have unless you engage in excessive worrying. I wondered if I had acted prematurely (yeah, right, after five years of dating*)*, or more importantly, if I had considered all the consequences and implications of getting married to Lynn. What would life be like in one, five, ten, or fifty years from now? I wanted a crystal ball to tell me what to do. No doubt, I was not heading in a useful direction when I started to think about fifty years into the future.

I did not want to subject her to my OCD. By that I mean that I loved her too much to see her worry about me. One person obsessing at a time is enough. *Oh, come on, I can't make someone else obsess! . . . . I know.* In addition, I did not know what the future would bring? Would I need hospitalization, like my friend in the support group, after his wife had a child? Would I be able to handle the stress that additional future responsibilities would bring? Would my OCD deteriorate and would she get stuck having to take care of me? Suddenly, these concerns and preoccupations surfaced. I had exerted no energy in regard to these thoughts at all in the past. Now a huge decision had to be made and swarming in the corners and crevices of my mind were scary and alienating thoughts.

I told her three or four months into our relationship that I suffered from OCD. She did not really know what that meant, but was open to talk about it. So, I educated her about my disorder. From time to time, I let her know what I reacted to in an anxious way (not what makes me anxious, nothing can make me anxious). She was aware that OCD was a part of my life and that with OCD comes ups and downs. *She always accepted me before, why would she change now? I don't know; it's just different. You're getting married! Masquerading as a "normal" person. Taking on the responsibilities of a husband and most likely a future father. Sometimes, I did not feel as if I could*

take care of myself, so how was I supposed to handle taking someone else's
needs into account too? Oh, come on. We've dated for a long time. I've done a
wonderful job as a boyfriend, why not a husband?

Lynn does many things that have helped me calm down when I'm
under OCD attack. First and foremost, she listens and doesn't judge me. She
tries to understand as well as a non-sufferer can. I might feel strange about my
thoughts or feelings, but after talking to her I feel like a regular human being
again. She experiences much of what I do, only to a lesser degree.

I remember arriving at her apartment one night when we were dating
and feeling distraught over an error that I had made at my first social work
internship. She listened, gave me a back rub, and lovingly stroked my brow.
She told me about some of the mistakes that she had made assisting people in
the intensive-care unit. She revealed some of the errors that other nurses had
committed on the job, some which could have had lethal consequences. She
said all the right and true things regarding mistakes -- everyone makes them,
and we can learn from them. Try not to commit the same mistake twice. Place
myself in others' shoes and then ask how I would feel and respond if somebody
did the same thing I did or said to them. Expand my perspective and envision
situations from different angles. If we shy away from making mistakes, we are
not fulfilling our potential as human beings. That very night, I knew that she
was the woman for me, she could comfort me and help me. I wanted and
needed her help the rest of my life. Lynn also helps me normalize what might
appear at first glance to be strange, bizarre behavior. My wife tells me that
sometimes she wants to wear a certain outfit so that she will have a good day.
Or that she wants to start and end on stairs with her right foot. We all perform
superstitious acts to make ourselves feel better and protect us against feeling
bad.

Spending a long time in front of the mirror in the bathroom, or
checking the front door, oven, or alarm clock more than once are pervasive
behaviors in our society. OCD takes it a little further, and sometimes a lot
further. However, everyone can relate to OCD on some level by scrutinizing his
or her current behaviors and habits. Individuals with OCD know that what they
are doing is absurd, silly, or unnecessary. They are no different than most
people, but their body and mind, for whatever reason, reacts differently to the
same, or a variation of the same, thoughts and behaviors that most people
experience. Anxiety seems to run the show. When you feel anxious, at least
you feel energized and are mobilized to ward off any danger. However, in the
back of your mind, you know the danger is not actually there. If the world
really was as dangerous as it seems to people with OCD, no one would be doing
anything and we would all have to lie in bed in the fetal position, prisoners of
our nervous systems and thoughts. It is a scary world at times for non-sufferers,
too. However, most people get along fine without worrying about all the things
that sufferers do.

Chapter 25

SELF-DISCLOSURE
AND THE REACTION OF OTHERS

After reading my parent's account of what transpired in the early years of my OCD, it reminded me of how secretive I had been about disclosing my diagnosis. A very painful, obsessional episode occurred at age sixteen when my friend and next-door neighbor discovered the journal that I was keeping that described my struggles with OCD. He saw only a few words, but I recall feeling completely defeated, violated, and lost. Someone had discovered the big secret. I had lost something and could never recapture the control I had over who knew and who didn't. I didn't want anyone to know because it all seemed so weird and abnormal. I didn't have any understanding about what was going on, so how could others?

The day of my friend's discovery, I remember going to the bank with my mother and telling her that I felt awful, not just awful, but really, really, awful. I didn't tell her why, but she already knew something was wrong. Lethargy and preoccupation invaded my being and the world was not right. I could not go on until there was some resolution to the matter.

Strangely enough, I never truly knew how much my friend had read. I knew that he said the word mental out loud, but at that point the book was closed. I had to explain the word mental, so I did the best that I could. I told him that I was writing about somebody else with mental problems. Nothing more was ever said. At any rate, my imagination created an entire scenario in which he did know everything about my problems and he would surely tell everyone. I was doomed. My fate had been decided. From then on, I would be known as the strange "mental" kid.

Of course, my imagination got the better of me, as it does with most individuals suffering from OCD. The uncertainty, the silence, and the fact that I saw this kid everyday conspired to remind me of that day. It seemed that life as it was before had changed and a new John bursted onto the scene. I detested this notion. I knew that life had not really changed and that the same John was still there. The only difference was that after my friend had happened upon my journal, I obsessed about that particular incident for a few months. It was one year after September 15, 1982, and that meant that my obsessions sometimes lasted for a significant period of time and became "distant" obsessions.

During high school, I wanted to keep my OCD to myself. No one could know about it; it was too bizarre. What would people think? I was already anxious enough. I didn't need more anxiety about how people judged me piled on to the old, regular, and everyday anxiety. I was not unlike most teenagers, I wanted to fit in, and I had a hard enough time doing it because I had problems and was quiet. I didn't need anything else getting in the way.

The one exception to the silence rule was my best friend Jake. It was very hard to even reveal myself to him, but my parents thought it might be a good idea. I was not sure why it was, but I agreed that he would be the easiest person to tell since we had gone through so much together. He could probably tell something was wrong anyway. One day after church, we got into a parked car. I told him that something important was on my mind and proceeded to describe my experiences as someone suffering from OCD. He took my disclosure in stride, as I knew a true friend would. The surprising thing to me was that after I told him I had OCD, he then disclosed some information about himself that was unknown to me up to that point. It's amazing how frequently secrets are kept from the best of friends. Even more astounding is to wonder how many other people have secrets about their life; some who may even be very close to you.

Though silence was usually the rule, I fantasized about telling my friends after I got out of high school. I think some part of me took pride in living with OCD and simultaneously performing very well in school. I didn't have green hair or play in a rock band, and I wasn't a great athlete or a Don Juan with the girls, but I **did** have OCD. It was a significant piece of my identity. The closer I got to graduation, the more coping with my OCD became "cool" in my mind. Graduation represented the end of a very important stage. I felt that maybe I could let peers in on my secret since we had spent the difficult and turbulent school years together. Since everyone would be going on to different colleges or other situations, it also felt less threatening to tell them this sensitive information.

Soon after my high school graduation, I started telling people. I walked into a retail store that one of my friends worked at and told him that I had OCD. I was surprised that he took the information in stride. It didn't seem like such a big deal anymore. *Hey, we made it through high school. Now I can tell people. Maybe they will even be interested in learning about OCD.* I was like a balloon that was popping. The pressure was unbearable and unrelenting. I knew that my emotional experiences in high school were not typical. I wanted to let everyone in on the secret. I had made it through school without anyone that I didn't want (except my neighbor) to know finding out. At this point in my therapy with my psychiatrist, we were discussing self-disclosure and meeting people. He suggested that when I met a girl, there were two things that I should not say: The first was, "Hi, my name is John, and I have OCD," and second, "Hi, I'm John. You have a great body." He had a good sense of humor and knew how to draw me out of myself. Because I trusted my therapist, I felt that he was giving me important tips that I took to heart.

After telling a few people, I became scared. I thought to myself, "What the heck am I doing? I don't want everyone and his brother to know. I realized that I told them on my own terms, but did I disclose to too many people and was it weird to let them know?" I suddenly realized that life continued after high school and that I wanted to keep my friends and not be treated any differently than before my disclosure.

I continued grappling with the idea of self-disclosure during the summer after I graduated from high school. I remember attending a dance at a local university with a high school buddy of mine. Also at the dance was a woman who had been the object of my first crush in elementary school. She had blossomed into a beautiful woman. Boy, even at a young age, I knew how to pick 'em. I didn't know her well at the time of the dance, for we hadn't seen much of each other for a couple of years. But each of us was aware of who the other was.

Anyway, as the night progressed, I finally got up the nerve to ask her to dance. She had been dancing with a couple of guys, and it didn't look like anything serious was going on between them. We said "hi" to each other, I asked her, and then she turned me down. She brushed me off with a quick parry, saying, "Oh, I'm tired of dancing" or something along those lines. At that point, I was so focused and honed in on dancing with her that the thought of actually talking to her averted my consciousness. I felt rejected and slumped back to tell the bad news to my buddy. The entire night revolved around getting her to dance with me. At that time, asking girls to go out with me or even dance with me seemed like a hunt and conquest situation. My fantasy life was working overtime, thinking about being with her on the dance floor, and spending time with her afterwards. It all came crashing down on me.

Then, my OCD symptoms picked up. Feeling embarrassed about the rejection, my thoughts started revving up -- negative thoughts of course. Back then, I didn't have the tools that I now possess to acknowledge what the anxiety-provoking situation was, label it, and rebut the negative, unreasonable, and irrational thoughts that were blowing around in my mind. My bubble had been burst, and self-doubt and uncertainty colored everything that I did. I wasn't interested in the fun anymore, even though there were plenty of other women to dance with and potentially meet.

As elaborated upon earlier in the book, at the dance I began to wonder about my sexuality. *I must be gay. Look at the way I'm walking. I'm walking slumped over and I'm so skinny and unmanly. No other woman in the entire place will find me attractive and interesting. My God, look at the way my wrist is laying over the top of the chair. Was that the leg of the table or my friend's leg? It must have been my friend's leg. Now he thinks I'm gay. Man, now I looked over at a guy for too long and he thinks something strange is going on.* My thoughts were coming at me, and created by my brain, at a rapid-fire pace. I couldn't keep up with it all.

I experienced my body becoming more rigid. For the rest of the evening I walked like a marcher in a band and chose my words very carefully. I was so cautious about what I said that I hardly said anything. Turning to my buddy, I told him that I wanted to leave. He seemed to be OK with this, so we left. He could tell something was wrong because he knew me well and friends can sense when something is not right. I was quiet and upset about what had (or hadn't) transpired at the dance.

When we made it back to his car, I told him what was bothering me. Not only that, then I told him about my OCD. He didn't know what it was, but he was very cool about it. He wasn't one to judge, criticize, or ridicule. For him, there was no stigma attached to the disorder. I was still the same guy that he knew growing up and going to school. That hadn't changed. I trusted him enough to tell him a "secret" that I normally did not tell people. My friend listened carefully as I explained that OCD was the reason why escaping the dance was the most palatable alternative at the time. He didn't understand, but that was OK. He was listening. That's all that he had to do. Our relationship didn't change because of my self-disclosure. It is always a judgment call -- to tell or not to tell. Real friends will be fine with it. Others may not.

The only time that an individual told me, outside of my support group, that ever telling other people might not be in my best interest was when an ex-girlfriend said so in 1988. We were on friendly terms and she was trying to be helpful. Like so many, she was wary of the negative connotations that a mental or emotional disorder carried. I respected her intelligence and knowledge of the social sphere, so I listened to her more than most. I became more cautious about revealing personal information. Some may be wondering if we broke up in the first place because she was aware that I was suffering from OCD. I don't think so. She simply liked another guy more than she liked me. OCD hadn't interfered with our relationship.

When I led an OCD support group, everyone weighed in with their opinion about the subject of self-disclosure. Some believed that it was better to tell no one, save a spouse. Others were much more open about it and discussed it with friends and others in the family. Everyone was interested in knowing how much to reveal for insurance purposes at work, and how much to tell an employer if you were in a position that was classified a "top security clearance" job. An ex-armed forces pilot claimed that he was thrown out of the service because of his disorder. Others claimed that no one understood and that family members neglected them and paid them no attention. Still, some felt that others blamed them for their disorder.

Why is society so afraid of emotional disorders? Naturally, hearing stories of raving-mad killers in the news doesn't help. Individuals suffering from OCD are far from crazy and are not dangerous to anyone. In fact, individuals who suffer from OCD are less likely to harm others and more likely to be conscientious about the impact of their behavior on others.

In the course of writing this book, getting it edited, and searching for a publisher, some people learned that I had OCD. Feeling more comfortable about revealing very personal information, and how to respond to others' inquiries, has resulted in a slow but steady discovery that others are not bothered by my diagnosis. In fact, it has tended to be a positive force for most relationships, bringing me closer to others. A few people read the manuscript and suggested changes. Barbara, who first edited the book, was a complete stranger and only a voice over the telephone until we met three years into the book writing process. It was a little awkward at first. She believed in my book and had already edited and helped another OCD book get published. It helped me that she was familiar with OCD and was very enthusiastic about my story.

The first time I met Barbara was at an annual professional conference for the Obsessive-Compulsive Foundation. She and I sat in a hallway near the lobby of the Marriot Hotel. We were reviewing her first impressions and editions to the manuscript. I felt ambiguous about our location, attempting to calm myself by saying, "Nobody is going to see or hear anything, so everything is alright." She began to speak out loud and I was imagining that everyone overheard what she was reading from the manuscript. I knew some sufferers there and some of my colleagues were present, too. I dreaded it, but I exposed myself to anxiety, thinking, "Maybe someone has heard something." I hated this uncertain statement about something that I did not want to happen. But there was nowhere else to go to do this and we wanted to get something accomplished. *Is that my boss? Did Barbara just say the word suicidal? No, that isn't my boss, but maybe someone can hear around the near corner. No, no, no. Most people are in one of the sessions now; the chances are low that someone I know will walk through this hallway. Well, I'm not sure. Isn't Jean staying in this hotel? I don't want everyone at work to know, too.* My anxiety elevated in part as a response to Barbara's intimate knowledge of my psychological past. I felt totally vulnerable to something she might say about me or my writing. I was an open book, both figuratively and literally. She had changed so much of my writing, too. Perhaps this was a sign that all the work that I had done was poorly written and expendable. More likely was my fear that she thought I was really, really weird.

At that time, besides the members of the support group, this was the only other person other than my wife, family, close friends, and my psychiatrists and therapists to know that I had OCD. I knew that it would be difficult to divulge all the very personal information, but I also knew that I needed professional assistance with the book. I had to allow her in on my "secret." *I better get used to others being aware of my diagnosis because I'm writing a tell-all book. I hope that at least ten people read the book and that I make it to the Jerry Springer show! Maybe a family member will throw a chair at me. Better yet would be Oprah. Come on, you know that you want people to buy the book and not read it.*

The next person found out about my OCD from an unlikely source, the telephone. I arrived home one day and had received a message on my telephone answering machine from Barbara. She stated that she needed to speak to me about chapter three of my book. My mother-in-law Kate was in the kitchen with me. I realized that she must have heard, especially since our kitchen could only fit one person comfortably. My wife must have felt as though she was in an airplane's bathroom when she cooked. It was really not that small, but you get the picture.

I did the only thing I could do. I ran away and joined the circus. No, no I didn't do that. People could guess what I was obsessing about at any particular time by asking me questions that I could respond "Yes" or "No" to. No, OK, I didn't do that. I stunned myself by telling her what the call was about. I didn't know what I was expecting her response to be, but I sure was glad that she had already known me for thirteen years. That made telling her a little easier. She was interested in the book and surprised that I had OCD. I worried that Kate might change the way she approached and spoke to me in the future. *Now, she's finding out who I really am. She's probably wondering if her daughter is happy and if her grandchildren are being taken care of and are safe. Wait! I'm projecting my thoughts and fears onto her. I tend to do this. I guess it's easier than facing them myself. She's reacting like she just found out from me how tall I was. It's no big deal. Really!!* Fortunately, Kate and her husband Bob have not treated me any differently since that day. She has always been very supportive and has encouraged me to write. Anxiety does make a mountain out of a molehill. I was very proud of myself for being assertive by telling her, answering her queries without any hesitation, reluctance, or shame that OCD was a part of me. Assertiveness, or telling people the way things really were, typically reduced my anxiety. A few colleagues at work know that I have OCD and that I am writing and trying to get a book published on the subject. I have revealed the most to my clinical supervisor. Since we spend an hour a week together reviewing cases, I have had more time to speak to her about my private life. She has helped me think about when to tell my clients that I have OCD, something that I do very infrequently. Over the years, she has assisted me with hundreds of cases and has provided much sage advice.

The next person to become aware of my OCD was my niece Tracy. She accidentally came upon some of my manuscript. I was at my brother Tom's house with the rest of my family celebrating a birthday. I planned to read some of the manuscript during the day and had left it on a couch for a minute, thinking that it would be safe from any curious eyes. It was turned over while I went to grab something to drink. Upon my return, Tracy was looking at the top page. She flipped the paper back over as I approached the couch. I could not believe that someone had seen it. I was upset since it seemed that I had taken enough precautions to ensure my confidentiality. I grabbed the manuscript, without saying anything, and spoke to my wife about what had just occurred. I was the most upset about what page she happened to see. It was the beginning of the book where I spoke regarding suicidal feelings. *Now she knows what a wacko her uncle is. She's going to tell everyone and see me differently. I'm her weird uncle.* During the get-together, all I could think about was what she may have seen. Consequently, I decided to take matters into my own hands and I told her what she had just seen; I told her that I had OCD and that I was writing a book about it. I figured that she already knew this anyways. She appeared unsurprised to find out this information. Her reaction was very calm and helpful. After two hours of feeling anxious and upset, my anxiety diminished and I was able to gain perspective about the circumstances. I knew that Tracy would eventually read the book because I was going to self-publish even if I could not find a publisher. I reasoned that she would likely ask my sister, her mother, about what she had read. And that it would be OK if she found out that I had OCD. I didn't care if all she knew was the name of the diagnosis. She might have known anyways. That same day, I handed over the manuscript to my father David to read and edit. He had published two books in the past and was an excellent writer (and would not cost me as much as a professional editor). After reading it, he knew a lot more about my OCD experiences and internal makeup than he had before. I was resigned to the fact that he was going to know some of my private thoughts, even some that I had expended much energy hiding over the years. *He is my father! I know that he is proud of me and accepts and loves me for who I am! He can help me write about my problems more eloquently than I can myself. Also, he has prior knowledge about some of my problems. That might make it a little easier to know that he is already aware of my OCD.* As with other family members who have also seen some of the book, he wanted the best for me and helped me as much as he could. My family encouraged me to continue the long, arduous process of getting the book written, edited, and published. Though we didn't talk much about the contents of the book, I did feel closer to my family, knowing that nothing had changed despite my anxiety about them discovering my perceived and real shortcomings. My perceptions changed during the series of steps I took writing the book; they are not shortcomings so much as tendencies and exaggerated feelings.

As a therapist, I have had to struggle with the question of whether I should reveal my diagnosis. I do not the vast majority of times. But there are times that appear ready-made for such a disclosure. I have pulled out my OCD wild-card and played it when I judged that it was the best thing to do for the client. That is the key. I can never divulge this information for the purposes of helping myself in any way; that is not the reason the client and I are in session together. I am there solely for him or her and I have to keep my needs out of my office. I get my needs met elsewhere. I speak to my wife if OCD surfaces or if I need an audience. In addition, my therapist, whom I see every week, helps me to maintain my emotional well-being. I remember the first time that I self-disclosed as a therapist. I was working with a ten year-old boy who perceived that people at his home environment did not understand OCD and the challenges that it presented to him. He meant that they did not appreciate his pain and only saw the overt symptoms, and not the internal war, for which he should have received a "Purple" Heart. Of course, family members could only see the external manifestations of OCD; this was not their fault. He was stating what I have frequently felt over the years. He wished that he had a "physical" disorder because people understand those. Everybody has experienced "physical" pain and has a reference point to aid in comprehending it. Moreover, there is no stigma attached to "physical" pain. A stigma exists only when the "physical" pain is believed to be caused by an emotional disorder.

An urge flooded me to tell the boy right then and there that we were brothers-in-arms. I was not prepared for this situation, though I had thought and talked about it with my supervisor. The feeling to rush to his aid and rescue him almost knocked me off my feet. *Maybe I should tell him. Maybe if he knows it will help him. He seems to be asking me to answer him by revealing that part of myself.* I turned my energies to balancing the probable positive and negative effects of telling this particular boy at this particular time and place.

I decided not to tell him right away because I was extremely ambivalent and felt emotionally vulnerable. Being aware of the oft-present overresponsibility theme, I chose to regroup and speak to others who could help me sift through my thoughts and feelings. I was very relieved that I followed that course of action since I had always planned to be cautious and conservative regarding my most personal data. What I was happiest about was that I had identified a time when I experienced insecurities about the effect that revealing would have, and that despite a strong impulse to self-divulge, I gave myself time to reassess the entire scene. I have improved in this area!

As I stated before, the client's needs and the foreseen clinical outcome are the determining factors in deciding whether to tell a client. In this case, after careful deliberation with other professionals, I chose to tell him. Putting aside my inclination to feel and do the overresponsible thing, my colleagues and I believed that the boy might be helped by my self-revelation. He had strongly expressed his feelings of isolation, much more so than the typical kid. I even asked him if it would help knowing a peer who suffered with the same condition. I could arrange sending an email or having a phone meeting with another kid who was roughly the same age and who experienced at least one or two similar types of symptoms. He said that he did not know anyone and was scared to meet another new person with the disorder. It did not appear that I would do any harm to our relationship if I told him. I had known him for three months and I believed that in the worst-case scenario, no harm would come to him. I followed Hippocrates advice; first, do no harm.

During our next session, I told him that I had experienced many OCD symptoms in the past. He did not react negatively or positively. He was a little curious about the specifics of my condition in the past and requested that I tell him some of my old symptoms. I explained that I never reveal that information. He stopped talking and then attempted some exposures. The subject never came up again, and he never did speak any more about his loneliness with the condition. Therefore, I believe it did make a positive impression on him and helped further the cause of his treatment. Subsequent to my disclosure, treatment did appear to be going slightly better. Moreover, he did more exposures that he had not done before.

I have found that most of the time, kids react well to the news. They wonder why I had not told them in prior sessions. Their parents are typically pleased that finally, there is someone who really, truly, and undeniably knows the disorder. Many families have unsuccessfully tried a few therapists before coming to see me. In working with anxiety-prone families and sufferers, it is reassuring to learn that the therapist is intimately knowledgeable about the experience of OCD. Everyone is already anxious regarding the client's condition; no one needs to be **more** anxious because he or she are unsure of the therapist's deep understanding and empathy. The majority of people with whom I have worked do not know anyone else that has told them about their OCD. Frequently, someone asks me how common OCD really is. I believe that in my office clients do not feel alone whether I divulge or not. A colleague once said to me, "We know that you possess the empathy that is required to help OCD sufferers." Someone understands the powerful, extraordinary, and unique experience with which he or she is struggling. Someone is aware of the "OCD moment-of-truth," when agonizing emotional distress competes with the awareness that performing a ritual will only serve to harden the resolve of the OCD. Furthermore, "the moment-of-truth" is a battle between peace and chaos. A glimpse of tranquility flutters in and out of the mind, making the decision more confusing to hold the line against OCD. At the same time, a glance at the despair felt after doing a ritual surfaces, too. It typically lasts no more than a couple of seconds, but it seems to take hours to compute all the factors involved and make a decision whether to ritualize.

During a session with any client, I tend to say that I appreciate the effort that he or she is expending to combat OCD. It is a horribly anxiety-provoking situation in which he or she finds him or herself. In addition, I wish that there was an easier way to treat OCD. But unfortunately, right now there is not a less difficult CBT strategy that is effective other than E/RP. I attempt to educate and support a client while I pronounce that it is up to him or her what the response to treatment will be. I state that it is true that OCD may make it more difficult for him or her to function; however, I gradually and methodically make it clear that it is he or she who controls his or her destiny. In short, I work hard trying to provide empathy. In response, clients, whether they know about my OCD or not, usually do what I recommend.

Clients who know more about me often realize why I do what I do as a therapist. The motive seems perfectly clear. I want to help others with a disorder that I know too much about. The profit motive diminishes and clients understand the reasons I have for doing therapy. His or her care is very important to me. I may acknowledge my OCD history to increase the probability that he or she will engage in an exposure. And when I say that I know how hard something is, there is an implicit and tacit mutual understanding that is palpable. Recently, a teenager declared that maybe he would follow in my footsteps and become a psychotherapist. This was very flattering to hear. My OCD has not been a hindrance in treating people. In fact, I believe it leads to a closer therapeutic relationship and better treatment outcomes.

DIAGNOSTIC CRITERIA FOR OCD (300.3)
(AS DEFINED BY THE DSM-IV)

A. Either obsessions or compulsions:
    1. Obsessions:
        a) Recurrent and persistent thoughts, impulses or images that are experienced at some time during the disturbance as intrusive and inappropriate and that cause marked anxiety or distress.
        b) The thoughts, impulses, or images are not simply excessive worries about real-life problems.
        c) The person attempts to ignore or suppress such thoughts, impulses, or images, or to neutralize them with some other thought or action.
        d) The person recognizes that the obsessional thoughts, impulses, or images are a product of his or her own mind (not imposed from without as in thought insertion).

    2. Compulsions:
        a) Repetitive behaviors (e.g., hand washing, ordering, checking) or mental acts (e.g., praying, counting, repeating words silently) that the person feels driven to perform in response to an obsession, or according to rules that must be applied rigidly.
        b) The behaviors or mental acts are aimed at preventing or reducing distress or preventing some dreaded event or situation; however, these behaviors or mental acts either are not connected in a realistic way with what they are designed to neutralize or prevent or are clearly excessive.

B. At some point during the course of the disorder, the person has recognized that the obsessions or compulsions are excessive or unreasonable. **Note:** This does not apply to children.

C. The obsessions or compulsions cause marked distress, are time consuming (take more than 1 hour a day), or significantly interfere with the person's normal routine, occupational (or academic) functioning, or usual social activities or relationships.

D. If another Axis 1 disorder is present, the content of the obsessions or compulsions is not restricted to it (e.g., preoccupation with food in the presence of an Eating Disorder; hair pulling in the presence of Trichotillomania; concern with appearance in the presence of Body Dysmorphic Disorder; preoccupation with drugs in the presence of a Substance Use Disorder; preoccupation with having a serious illness in the presence of Hypochondriasis; preoccupation with sexual urges or fantasies in the presence of a Paraphilia; or guilty ruminations in the presence of Major Depressive Disorder).

E. The disturbance is not due to the direct physiological effects of a substance (e.g., a drug of abuse, a medication) or a general medical condition.

With poor insight: Occurs when a sufferer, for most of the time during the current episode, does not recognize that the obsessions and compulsions are excessive or unreasonable.

American Psychiatric Association: *Diagnostic and Statistical Manual of Mental Disorders*, Fourth Edition. Washington, DC, American Psychiatric Association, 1994.

REFERENCES

I hope that our time together has increased your understanding of OCD. Though there is much information in this book, I would be remiss if I didn't also provide information about some helpful resources from the OCD community.

1) Obsessive-Compulsive Foundation, Inc.
676 State St.
New Haven, CT 06511
Phone: (203) 401-2070
Fax: (203) 401-2076
E-mail: info@ocfoundation.org
Website: www.ocfoundation.org

The OC Foundation can provide referrals in your area. As a member, you receive a valuable and informative newsletter. In addition, they maintain an extensive list of books, pamphlets, audiotapes, and videotapes.

2) Anxiety Disorders Association of America (ADAA)
8730 Georgia Ave. Suite 600
Silver Spring, MD 20910
Phone: (240) 485-1001
Fax: (240) 485-1035
Website: www.adaa.org

The ADAA can assist with referrals to professionals and support groups. It also offers resources of all different types.

3) OC Information Center

Madison Institute of Medicine
7617 Mineral Point Rd., Suite 300
Madison, WI 53717
Phone: (608) 827-2470
Fax: (608) 827-2479
E-mail: mim@miminc.org

The Center is the best source of popular and professional articles about OCD. You can also order printouts of computer searches on specific OCD topics.

4)   National Institute of Mental Health (NIMH)
     Neuroscience Center (NSC) Building
     6001 Executive Boulevard
     Rockville, MD 20852
     Website: www.nimh.gov

The NIMH has done, and may be currently conducting, much valuable and important research about OCD. In addition to being a great source of up-to-date information on OCD, you can also request information about different research protocols in which you may be able to participate.

383 #

86 1/.

S. Nauk.

Suring